PATERSON, John K.

Who'd be a patient?

WHO'D BE A PATIENT?

WHO'D BE A PATIENT?

John Paterson

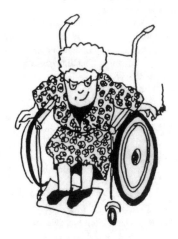

Book Guild Publishing
Sussex, England

First published in Great Britain in 2008 by
The Book Guild Ltd
Pavilion View
19 New Road
Brighton
BN1 1UF

Typesetting in Times by
IML Typographers, Cheshire

Printed in Great Britain by
CPI Antony Rowe

A catalogue record for this book is available from
The British Library.

ISBN 978 1 84624 261 8

For those who may have 'been there' – though perhaps not by choice.

Contents

Preface

Why on earth should anybody want to read this book? Surely it is bad enough being a patient, without adding to the agony by reading about it? Why should other people's problems be of the slightest interest? The last question is easy to answer. They might well reflect your own but, of much greater value, you might find them amusing or even a comfort. On what authority is the book written, anyway? The answer to that is long experience – of being both doctor and patient. I know which rôle I prefer.

Being a patient is not necessarily agonising, although it is often something of a bore, and it may also affect others in various ways and to varying degrees. In fact, there are patients who actually enjoy their sorry state. One of the interesting things about being a patient is that the word implies someone who suffers – and after all, sympathy means suffering with someone else. Sharing the burdens of sickness and sorrow is certainly therapeutic – why not also share the laughter? That could prove therapeutic, too.

Perhaps you have been brain-washed into thinking of yourself as a somewhat impersonal 'client', or possibly a 'user' of an institutionalised service. Whether or not that is the case, experiencing the state for yourself can still be funny. And this is something you may learn to share – sometimes laughing at the more entertaining episodes in other people's lives, and in return giving them the giggles over some of your own unplanned experiences. It is this laughter that often makes the patient's agony less, and may also reduce the effects on others. So the answer to the second question is pretty obvious.

I have good cause to write this small book. Like many boys, I first learned to laugh at adversity at school, being rather small and very short-sighted from an early age. I found nothing funny about boxing – I could not see what I was meant to be hitting, let alone what was coming my way. And I did not much care for the school doctor sewing up my scalp after injury on the rugby field. But otherwise I managed to steer clear of the medical profession for the whole of my school days – other than for routine weighing and measuring and the odd 'jab'. The rest of my early learning to laugh was not as a patient – it was in the usual adversarial contacts with other boys.

I built on this minor educational base during the second world war, when I discovered that laughing at some of the horrors and trials of warfare was almost literally life-saving. Some of those tales are to be found elsewhere – and I survived almost unscathed.

After the war I returned to my interrupted studies, and once I had qualified, I went on to working hideously long hours in hospital, where laughter kept us going remarkably well. Then, after a brief spell in an inner-city practice in London, I had the enormous privilege of working as a family doctor in a scattered rural community – my average weekly hours plummeted from ninety-six to a modest sixty-eight. And I still found great comfort in being able to laugh, not at my patients but with them.

My greatest authority to write this book came later – I became a serious patient myself. It was only then that I fully learned about the problems of 'patienthood' – and to laugh about them even more. I have to tell you that every one of the tales here is based on real live fact. But it is well to remember that they mostly come from a time when the doctor–patient relationship was rather different from that often found in today's demanding, administration-ordered, litigation-driven, defensive medical supermarket. In both my roles I am seriously concerned as to how the service has evolved and what we may best do for the future.

I am deeply grateful to Alison Frances for capturing the spirit of the book in her charming sketches.

JOHN PATERSON

1

First Weeks as a Doctor

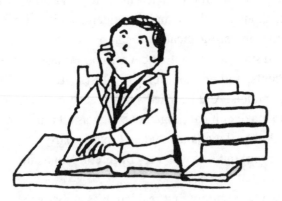

Even for an old soldier who thought he had learned how to communicate with people, the realisation that I was at last qualified as a doctor was quite something to take in. For a start I had doubts about my reading ability. I had to go back to the notice board outside the Senate House of the University of London to make sure it really was my number that I thought I had read on the crucial pass list – was it 321 or 312 I had seen? The magic number was there – a short holiday with my wife and two small children was clearly indicated. Two small children as a medical student? Yes indeed, but you have to remember that I was six and a half years older than most of my contemporaries. In fact several of the ex-service students had families. What mattered was that I had made it at last. We had earned a short break.

The same evening any such hopes were dashed. The head of the Obstetric Department rang in person to ask me to do a locum job for him, as Junior Obstetric House Physician, starting the following morning. So much for our little holiday. In the event, that holiday was deferred for a number of years, but first things first.

Of course, a houseman is a dogsbody but, accepting that, he is also in a prime position for learning. My first day was one long surprise, though without major incident. I played a very minor role in the operating theatre, accompanied the chief on a ward round, and survived an outpatient session. At last I was seeing real live patients, rather than for the most part carefully selected teaching models. And I carried a tiny measure of responsibility – I started to make clinical judgements. It was all rather sobering. We had had lots of laughs as students (particularly amongst the ex-service group) but this was very different. Not a single laugh was to be heard that first day.

Day two brought my first real laugh as a doctor. My chief had a patient in his outpatient clinic who had a complicated blood problem, so he very properly sought advice from his old friend, the head of Haematology. Like my chief, he was a Yorkshireman. George, the worthy haematologist, duly appeared in the clinic, where he looked at the patient, discussed the diagnostic possibilities and advised on what should be done. After his consultation, he was invited to have a cup of tea in Sister's office together with my chief, the obstetric registrar, the nurse dealing with the patient in the clinic, and me. Sister's room in the old hospital was very small, and there was not room for the assembled company to sit – there were no more than two chairs for six behinds. Nonetheless, some quite tasty buns were offered, and soon each one of us had a cup and saucer in one hand and a small plate in the other. I kept very much in the background.

The technical problem out of the way and the blood sample in the haematologist's pocket, out of the blue my boss asked his visitor whether he knew about the three stages of growing old. Old George shook his head thoughtfully.

'No.'

'Well, George, I really thought you would have known. But no. So I suppose I shall have to tell you. In the first stage you keep forgetting people's names.'

'Aye.' Head on one side, he waited for his host to continue.

'In the second stage you forget to do up your flies after you've been for a pee.'

'Aye.' Our guest looked distinctly puzzled. What on earth had this to do with a rare corner of haematology – or with obstetrics? 'Go on, then. Let's have number three.'

'In the third stage you forget to undo your flies in the first place.'

'Aye.' He shook his head in total incomprehension, while the rest of the assembled company awaited our chief's next comment. His facial expression told us nothing.

'Eh, George, you're in the second stage.'

There stood our guest, aghast, his hands occupied with cup and plate, Sister's small desk out of reach, while we all dissolved into laughter. Happily no patients were there to witness this frivolity, but it certainly set the scene for the rest of my short time in that delightful unit.

The very next day I was to be involved in a further amusing incident – this time involving a patient rather more intimately. My task was to do the weekly 'ring clinic'. Still situated in the wartime basement of the old hospital, the clinic was equipped with eight beds, curtained off from each other, with a sink for scrubbing up between each. Our job was the routine change of the pessaries of elderly ladies of the locality who were unfit for the harsher alternative of surgery. Not the pleasantest of tasks, but necessary. Working rather fast, I got ahead of 'my' nurse, starting on an elderly lady already installed on a bed and prepared for the procedure. As I was struggling to remove the old pessary, the patient suddenly grasped my left wrist with a claw-like hand.

'Not very pretty down there, are we, doctor?'

I had certainly not expected anything like this and I fear my immediate response was not entirely appropriate.

'That all depends on your point of view.'

The grip on my wrist tightened, as I called for the nurse to rescue me. Happily, my patient released me with a giggle. I certainly never made that mistake again.

Soon after, I spent my first weekend as a doctor at a small women's hospital, so as to allow the resident medical officer to have a well-earned couple of days off. There was no routine work involved; I was to be there just in case of emergency on the wards. In fact I had nothing at all to do on the Friday night. On the Saturday morning, a rather urgent surgical operation had been arranged, to be performed by a well-known visiting surgeon, Mr Leary. Knowing him to have something of a reputation technically, I asked Matron whether she thought I might be allowed to come to theatre to watch. She told me to ask him, and at that moment he emerged from his very elegant Rolls Royce and strode through the door. He was a small man, very quick in everything he said or did, sporting a strong Irish accent. I had no difficulty in taking Matron's advice. His immediate response was straightforward enough.

'My dear fellow, there's no point in gawping. I'd be delighted if you would assist.'

This was great. On my arrival in theatre, the patient was already anaesthetised. It was immediately made clear that my role was not to be hovering in the background, observing things – the great man certainly expected me to be an active member of the team. And he worked very fast – but astonishingly precisely. I just had to comment on his high-speed technique. I was very concerned that the poor patient seemed to be awash with blood, so I cautiously questioned Mr Leary about the considerable amount of bleeding that was taking place. His immediate response was something of a surprise.

'Oh, it doesn't matter if the whole pelvis is full of blood. She's got plenty going in, and we can always mop the mess up afterwards.'

I was glad the patient was unconscious at the time. She might have been a trifle taken aback to have heard that. The bold surgeon was quite right in what was to happen – she did have an ample supply going in, we did mop her up afterwards. And later on that day, when I visited her on my routine round, I found her in remarkably good shape.

Some weeks later the young man whose job I had taken over for the weekend finished his six-month stint there and threw a small farewell party. He very kindly invited me. Yes, the 'bloody' surgeon was there, too – with his delightful Irish wife. Towards the end of that party, my young host pressed Mrs Leary to have another drink.

'Oh, no thank you, Andrew, no alcohol – just a little gin.'

The next week found me in a sector hospital, as a locum house surgeon to the plastic surgery unit. This I found fascinating. Some miles to the south of London, the hospital occupied a number of huts scattered over a large compound which had been a military base of some sort for much of the war. It was not a very welcoming place and, November being upon us, it was quite chilly between wards. The resident staff numbered six: two registrar grade doctors, one surgical, the other medical, one anaesthetic houseman, one medical houseman and two surgical housemen. Of the latter, one dealt with ear, nose and throat problems and the female general surgical patients, while the other served the plastic surgery unit and looked after the male general surgical patients. This small group was very different from the hordes of people in my teaching hospital. Oh, and for some reason we also had a very pleasant resident padre. Various senior staff visited us from time to time. There were few dull moments, and I quickly learned a great deal about the nitty-gritty of medical practice, but one episode was truly unforgettable.

It was a lovely Saturday afternoon, and I wished I could have been out walking. But I was on call, so I was quietly reading one of the several medical journals in the soulless common room. I was in the middle of a fascinating report on resuscitation when the telephone rang – the caller was one of the local GPs. He was charming, apologising for troubling me on a Saturday afternoon, and asking me if I could see a small boy who had 'cut his head a bit'. As a budding plastic surgeon, I was delighted at this opportunity to do a bit of sewing up. The only hitch was that only two of the medical staff were on site at the time. The surgical registrar and the medical houseman were on leave for the weekend, the medical registrar was out visiting a sick nurse in her lodgings, and the anaesthetic houseman had walked down to the nearby town to go to the cinema. That left the other house surgeon and me.

We did not have long to wait. When the small patient arrived, I was horrified to find that his injury was a bit more than I had understood. The history I had been given was not really full

6

enough. His parents soon put me right – he had fallen off a ten-foot high wall onto cobble-stones. Harry's scalp was split from close to one eye to well behind his ear, with the free part flapping out like a wing. With the edges held together, the cut was seven inches long. Cut his head a bit! He was conscious, but confused. Clearly I had to exclude bony injury, so before anything else, he needed to be X-rayed. With no radiographer on duty I had to do this myself – my first ever skull X-ray! I managed to get the positioning right, largely by chance I made a suitable choice with regard to exposure time, and went on to develop the plate. It was a gratifyingly good picture, but I was horrified by what I saw. I was uncertain about the bony appearance close to where he had hit the cobbles. Had he a fracture, or not? How much brain damage might underlie it?

I called Kevin, the ENT houseman (who had six months more experience as a doctor than I), who assured me that the odd appearance was normal for a boy of Harry's age. Kevin agreed that I should do the necessary sewing, and that he would give the anaesthetic, but we were unaware that the lad had not long before had an enormous lunch. Yes, soon after the start of being anaesthetised, he vomited profusely. There was vomit every-where. On the operating table, on the floor, in Kevin's lap and filling the anaesthetic mask. There was nothing else to do but to pack up, mop up and try again an hour later. This we had to explain to Harry's anxious parents. Happily they accepted our advice very readily.

In the end we triumphed. Kevin was more successful with his second attempt to anaesthetise the lad, and I put in thirty-two stitches – I thought jolly well. He certainly looked a lot tidier. And then the anaesthetic houseman returned from the cinema.

'Have you two been having fun?'

We could have throttled him. And, to make matters worse, he went on to say that the film he had been to see was excellent.

Of course, to be on the safe side I had to admit Harry to hospital, and the next morning, after a rotten night of worry, I nipped along to the ward before breakfast, rather dreading what I might find. Harry was up and about, positively chirruping, helping the staff to distribute tea and toast to bed-ridden patients. His wound looked fine. He was in great form, so I sent him home very pleased with himself – an expert ward assistant. I seriously considered taking up plastic surgery – the fiddliness of it all appealed to me greatly, and I only decided against this after considering the weight of unnecessary cosmetic surgery. I could never have coped with that. No, this sort of thing was what plastic surgery ought to be about – mending patients who had suffered accidental injury. No surgical stuffing and slimming for me, thank you.

Another memorable episode stays with me. We did a very complicated job on a man who had been involved in a horrific traffic accident. Apart from gross facial damage, his jaw was shattered. So my boss had arranged for a professor of dental surgery to take part in a joint undertaking – he was to fix the jaw in good alignment, while we were to go on to put a face round his work, a two-part operation. I was so impressed with Professor Tinker that, after the operation, I asked him if he could advise me on my dental state. Though I had never had toothache in my life, I had not seen a dentist for seven or eight years. I saw him a few days later and he did some very basic repair work. More than half a century later I have had three of his repairs 'patched' and still do not know what toothache feels like. What a good thing I did that brief plastic surgery job.

At Christmas we had some harmless fun. As Father Christmas,

the surgical registrar was installed on a surgical trolley as a sledge, suitably decked out with a scarlet hospital blanket. The medical houseman was the front half of the towing reindeer, the back half being the resident anaesthetist. Where they had got their peculiar costume from I do not remember, but instead of antlers it had a trunk! I borrowed a tutu from one of the nurses, to be an attendant fairy. It was far too small, but I managed to get it laced up behind, and I carried a large wooden spoon as my fairy wand. We were a great success with the patients, but it was damned cold between wards.

After seven wonderful weeks in the post, I went back to my old hospital for six months' slog as a casualty officer. No more airy walks between one job and another – this was back to the tunnel-like corridors of a Victorian medical palace, leading to unimaginable 'action stations' on every hand. Behind almost every door there was a surprise lurking.

2

Who'd be a Casualty Officer?

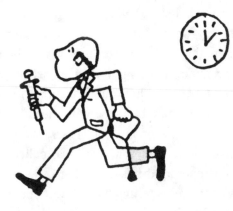

In the old days, before Casualty had for some unaccountable reason been re-labelled Accident and Emergency, it fell to the hospital porters to do a great deal of informal selection of patients turning up at the hospital unannounced. While it might have caused a few administrative frowns, in practice this worked very well. The porters were all locals, who knew the inhabitants of the area well – including the regular customers – and who also understood the problems facing the professional staff of the department. They made it their business to get to know each new bunch of casualty officers, and they were an immense help to us, at times channelling patients to particular members of staff in a wholly informal, yet highly effective way. And they occasionally gave us valuable advice about individual patients – the 'regulars'.

It was quite an eye-opener. Eight of us juniors worked under two rather more senior doctors, the Resident Medical Officer and the Resident Surgical Officer, manning the very busy department in shifts twenty-four hours a day. We called for specialist help as required. Literally anything might come through those doors, or so it seemed, and at any time of the day or night. And, of course, it included the inevitable Saturday night drunks. By the time I arrived for my six-month stint in the department, the porters already knew that I had ended the war as a junior officer in the Army Commando, returning to medical school after my six-and-a-half-year sabbatical. Their interpretation of this was that I was probably better prepared to cope with these sometimes awkward characters than some of my colleagues who had come straight from school. So they saw to it that I was called upon to deal with the more obstreperous drunks, whether I was officially on duty or not. I do not remember telling them that at one time I used to teach unarmed combat, but this seemed unnecessary – I got called out just the same. And I really enjoyed it – most of the time.

One Saturday night episode sticks in my mind. A particularly noisy and violent drunk staggered into the department shortly after closing time, causing considerable disturbance. In line with their unofficial practice, the struggling porters installed him in one of the eight small examination rooms and sent for me (although I was technically off duty). When I arrived from my room just across the road, they just stood back and let me get on with the job. This particular patient proved quite a problem to cope with and, in the course of my somewhat physical encounter with him, he managed to kick me in the face. I did not suffer any real harm, but my specs were shattered. Being very short-sighted, I was rendered completely *hors de combat*.

It was only then that I realised what an ass I was. Throughout the war, both at home and in my several journeyings in India and Burma, I had made a point of carrying a spare pair of specs. In spite of a sometimes chaotic life, I had never needed them. Now, in the heart of London, I was incapable of doing my job – I was a casualty myself. And it was largely my fault. Feeling something of a clot, I rang my wife Mary in Wimbledon, asking her to find someone to look after the children while she brought me my spare pair, thirteen stops on the District line. This was a great start to my term in the post.

What was it I had heard about the importance of the doctor–patient relationship? Happily it was not all like that. But what was certain was that, in such a department, there was no limit to what might happen. Very late one evening one of the staff midwives called in, seeking a houseman to accompany her to a home delivery somewhere in Battersea. The other midwife on duty had already gone out in the company of the obstetric house physician, and now there was another call. Mrs Ivers was said to be well advanced in labour in a council flat, some way from the hospital. I was more than happy to oblige. This would be my first home confinement and I really relished the sense of doing something vicariously creative.

First we had to go down to the basement to collect a couple of bicycles, as there was no car available – there was only one 'district' car, and of course it was out on the previous job. As we emerged from the basement into Central Hall, two policemen appeared at the entrance, asked us where we were going, and firmly told us to leave the bicycles where they were, it would only waste time to put them away now. Where was it we wanted to go? Battersea – no problem. They would give us a lift to the door. We were whisked away in great style, screeching through Lambeth at an exciting rate, to save time even going the wrong way along a one-way stretch, just beyond the foot of Lambeth Bridge. In a very few minutes we were dropped at the block of flats which was our destination. We would have to take the tram back in the morning, but no matter.

Mrs Ivers was an old hand, her previous two children both having been born at home. She was indeed well into the second stage of labour, having very strong contractions. I was to do the delivery, the relatively experienced midwife discreetly supervising me. The bedroom was perfectly adequate and spotlessly clean, but Mrs Ivers' bed was very low. After a quick wash I found that I had to kneel down to get to grips with the job. This did not worry me at all – I could do a lot worse than kneel. A short while later, the midwife encouraged me to restrain the infant's head, to avoid damage to the mother from a too-rapid delivery. I did as I was told – of course.

Or I thought I did. Then I noticed something rather odd – the infant's head seemed to be getting further away from me, as my arms stretched out more and more. The cause of this was soon apparent – the force of the mother's contractions worked intermittently to make the infant's head advance, while my restraining push, far from being very effective, resulted in me travelling across the polished linoleum of the bedroom floor on my knees. Jolly good contractions they were too, if they could propel me about the room. Well done, Mrs Ivers.

The infant duly arrived, mum needed not even the tiniest repair, and she joined in the laughter over having literally pushed the doctor around at our first meeting. I do not suppose she ever forgot that night – it certainly remains with me. What a way to start my long list of home confinements. The midwife and I packed our bags and took the tram back to hospital, in time for me to put the unused bicycles back in the basement and go back to work in Casualty for the last hour or so of my shift.

One of the interesting things about this job was that it was essentially a learning post. Anything of particular interest was likely to be seen by all of us currently on duty. Of course, this led to some delays for patients, but it was well worthwhile, for them as well as for us, as we could discuss our findings with each other, or with the more senior chaps. Again and again the 'old soldiers' found communication with patients much easier than did the 'schoolboy' doctors amongst us. This held advantages for us and for the patients, who found themselves talking to more adult people. But it made me wonder why on earth we had been taught so very little about the matter of communication with patients while we were undergraduate students. It would have helped the youngsters enormously.

A diagnostic rarity was an indication for the appropriate specialist to be called down to the department to give advice. Two cases stand out in my mind. One day we were all told to down tools and come to a particular cubicle – a rather large lady needed sorting out. She was in her late forties, quite a bit overweight, with pain high up in her tummy on the right side. The consultant told me to take a history and examine her. The story suggested possible gall bladder disease, but I pummelled about for a while without really making any diagnostic decision. I could not be sure of what I felt. Two more casualty officers had a look before we left the good lady with the nurses to discuss the case out of earshot.

'Well, Paterson, I think you got the history all right. What did you find on examination?'

'To be honest, Sir, I couldn't make head or tail of it. There was rather a lot of fat about, nothing seemed clear-cut. What could you actually feel, Sir?'

His reply was a joy to hear.

'You might as well palpate a bolster. A clinical diagnosis is impossible – the patient needs further investigation. We'll get on with that now.'

I have had visions of bolsters on numerous occasions since. Just show me a lass with a pain in her tummy who is fair, fat and forty, and I start to laugh. And laughing assists memory very well.

Another case was very different. A most rare skin condition had presented. We gathered round, waiting for the words of wisdom. The dermatologist was already there. The patient was a young man who looked pretty fit, if a bit embarrassed by the attention he was getting. All he had was an odd-looking open sore on the back of one hand, which we all had to look at with care. It did not seem to us to be of great significance. Maybe six weeks was rather a long time for him to have had it, but it did not look very different from what one might expect a sore hand to look like. Then we were let into the secret – it was a cattle ringworm. This was a great rarity, and we would be unlikely to see it again in our professional lives. The patient was a little taken aback by all the fuss over his sore hand, and he was adamant that he had never touched a cow in his life – or not a four-legged one, he added.

I forget what treatment he was afforded or how well it worked. But I was later to find that it was by no means a rare condition – within a year or so I was seeing one case every few weeks in rural general practice. I suppose that one was not likely to see such a patient in a London teaching hospital – infected cattle were not prone to wander the streets of Lambeth. But this did not mean that the condition was rare – what it demonstrated very clearly was the fact that a London teaching hospital sees but a very small percentage of what goes wrong in the great wide world, and that what it does see is highly selected.

This encounter reminds me of a sequel to it, some years later. I saw a case of cattle ringworm in a farm worker from an outlying hamlet. I had seen quite a few before, and by this time I knew the practice area and some of its inhabitants quite well. I had always enjoyed driving about the countryside with my eyes open. Always a lover of the outdoor life, I habitually observed a lot of detail on my rounds. One of the things which struck me was that none of the cases of cattle ringworm I had seen came from farms where fences were regularly creosoted. The likely answer had to be that, to reduce the itching, cattle with early ringworm rubbed themselves on the fences. If those fences had been recently creosoted, the cattle got traces of creosote on their skin. I had never come across cattle with ringworm in fields bounded by recently creosoted fences.

So yes – I bought a small quantity of crude creosote in the neighbouring town, made up an ointment by simply stirring some of it into the standard ointment base, and sent the farm worker off to apply it twice a day. Not very accurate dosage perhaps (I made no attempt to measure how much I added – I just thought the colour looked all right). Within days he was completely cured. So that became a therapeutic habit in the practice. Some months later I met our local dermatologist and I told him of my success with some pride. He was horrified, even when I reassured him that my success rate was one hundred percent.

That is jumping the gun a bit. Back in Casualty I saw my first case of attempted suicide. It was a horrid shock to me, even though I had seen some pretty nasty injuries during the war. I was disturbed that this young woman should have reached such a level of despair. She had slashed both wrists with a razor blade and was bleeding seriously. Of course, while I sewed her up and bandaged her wrists I talked to her. Nellie objected strongly to my efforts, insisting that she had made up her own mind on the matter and that she had every intention of doing it again at some later date. Nothing I said made any difference, and I was left wondering how I was helping.

This was my first experience of the problem – but not my last. And it made me think of the wider family problems around death from whatever cause. I remembered the real difficulty I had found in writing to the parents of one of my troop who had been killed in action. Two total strangers to be offered the agonising truth about their son. That letter had taken me a long time to write.

Returning from a rare weekend off duty one morning, I emerged from Westminster underground station to find crossing the road impossible. The Westminster Bridge traffic kept coming, the Whitehall and Parliament Square traffic was non-stop, both streams competing for precedence at the junction with the Embankment. I was going to be late – something I could never countenance. It was my grandmother who had taught me always to be 'ten minutes punctual'. Then, quite suddenly, London came to a grinding halt. A large blue figure strode across from the traffic island where he was on point duty, took me by the arm and marched me to the other side of the road – while London waited.

'Never thought I'd see you 'ere, Sir. I 'ope I'll see you at the reunion.'

With that he went back to his traffic island and started London up once more. I went to work, having a quiet laugh as I went. I had last seen him as a member of my troop in No. 1 Commando in Burma.

In Casualty they still kept coming. The doors seldom remained closed for more than a few minutes. Not long after the traffic episode another odd thing happened. As the official hospital for the Metropolitan Police, we saw a number of these chaps every day. They used to call in sometimes for a cup of coffee with the porters, while at other times they would bring in the survivor of a traffic accident or a delinquent in need of medical help. They were very much 'part of the furniture'.

On this occasion two of these large, blue men appeared, for no apparent reason. It was only a moment before I recognised one of them – yes, it was the chap on point duty who had rescued me from London's traffic. Stan Barber had been unofficial troop funny man towards the end of the war, keeping us all in fits of laughter. Neither of us was a patient this time, but we met up again after work that evening in Rochester Row Police Station, where I was royally entertained until some ungodly hour. He had made us laugh in Burma, and he had certainly not lost any of this ability on coming back to civilian life. Of course, the cockney funny man is always very funny. I am sure he kept laughing to the end of his days.

Apart from the chap who kicked me in the face and the lass who objected to my mending her self-inflicted wounds, I had nothing but gratitude from the multitude of patients I saw. The ongoing toil of Casualty continued, and this raises an interesting point. Many people think that very long hours of work are dangerous, in that one is more likely to make mistakes when tired. While there must be some truth in this, far more important is that what is most tiring about long hours is boredom. Working in Casualty there is no room for boredom. Every time one sees a new patient one 'changes gear' in communicating with a fresh individual and in dealing with a different problem. Every patient presents a fresh challenge, and this demands that the doctor automatically rises to the occasion – and the chance of a laugh is considerable. In this exciting six months my average working week was ninety-six hours. It was a wonderful experience.

3

In at the Deep End

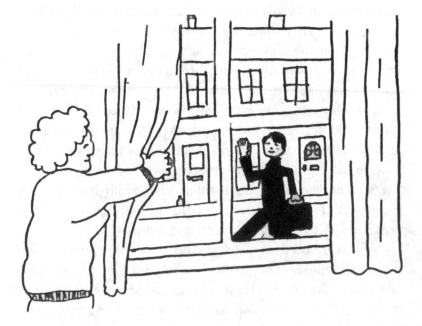

After six months in Casualty I was ready to move on. I had been appointed house surgeon to the senior consultant surgeon in the hospital but, in spite of Mary's clearly voiced disapproval, I had decided against taking up the post. The reason for this was entirely economic. A consultant post was at best seven years away, more likely ten, and my gross pay was three hundred and fifty pounds a year – fifty pounds a year *less* than my ex-service educational grant had been. Increases in pay over the next seven to ten years were likely be pretty modest, and I had no resources other than what I earned. With a family to support I found it immoral to go ahead with any personal aspirations, when I could double my income overnight and probably treble it within the year. It was great to have been appointed to the job, but I just could not bring myself to take it up. I made history by resigning one of the two most coveted junior posts in the hospital.

A further matter concerned me – I had been seeing a great variety of patients and problems in Casualty, but they all came from an inner-city background, and they had almost all been selected as suitable teaching material. I had a feeling that things in a more relaxed community might be very different. But I was certainly not yet ready for the 'big move'. So I chose to take a six-month trainee post in general practice in Paddington, before moving on. One of the chief attractions of this was that I could live with my family for the first time since qualifying. This was the moment for me to start on a further learning curve. It was to prove very different from the last few months.

The surgery occupied a small shop in the High Street. Inside there was a tiny entrance lobby with an inner door to a staircase and a second door on the right to what had been the front half of the shop. The original shop window made it an extremely light room – this was the waiting room. Apart from a few chairs and a table heaped with out-of-date magazines, the room was adorned with a most sensible notice for anxious young mothers: 'The food your child doesn't eat never does him any harm.'

I found this notice delightful. While simple, it was so profound. Too much rot is talked and written about child nutrition. And adult nutrition for that matter. As a result of this too many mothers are needlessly worried when nature tells their children they have had enough. Except for poverty-stricken areas, there are many more obese children in this world than skinny ones. And obesity is a very serious matter. But I thought we needed one more notice about diet – warning against stuffing oneself with unnecessary, unhealthy foodstuffs. More of that later.

Otherwise there was nothing notable about the waiting room – it was clean, there were a few pictures on the walls, some of them advertising material from drug manufacturers – it was just typically uninteresting. Patients let themselves in and sat down, and waited for the doctor to come and fetch them, when he saw his previous patient out. And this revealed a very pleasant courtesy on the part of the doctors, in that they habitually welcomed patients in and ushered them out in person. Not always the practice today. This small gesture seemed to me very much a part of the very important 'doctor–patient relationship' and conducive to a high quality of service.

The second door to the waiting room opened into a dark little passage, from which there were three more doors. On the right there was a tiny consulting room, with no natural lighting, while at the far end there were two rather larger consulting rooms, each with a very modest window onto the small yard behind the shop. Mavis occupied the flat upstairs and did the cleaning and some simple secretarial chores in the evenings, mainly filing. She had no contact with patients.

There was one very odd feature of the set-up. Above desk level the two large consulting rooms were separated by a large bank of two-sided pigeon-holes – accessible from either side. This was where patients' records were kept, so that either of the two partners had immediate access to them. The notes were in alphabetical order, so they ran from left to right, from top to bottom in one room, but from right to left in the other. Of course this arrangement limited privacy, but in practice it did not really matter as, due to outside commitments, the two partners were virtually never in their rooms at the same time. And, having no secretary/receptionist (other than the worthy Mavis), it was very convenient to have such ready access to records. Nonetheless on very rare occasions it could be quite unnerving for a patient to hear a rustle and see notes being tweaked out from the other side.

The little dark room was mine, but of course I had to have a record card given to me with each patient. This extended the atmosphere of courtesy very agreeably. My tutor, Charles, was a quiet, gentle man, with a natural bent for teaching. He would introduce me to each patient, hand me the card and leave me to get on with the job. He could not have been more helpful to me. With no commitment to emergency or night work (and for the first time in more than eight months living at home with my family) I started work at nine each morning. On finishing with each patient I ushered him or her out, and reported to Charles when he next showed a patient out. He would then introduce me to my next patient. This continued until nearly lunch time. Then I would take along my accumulated records, and the two of us would sit down together in his room and discuss every patient I had seen that morning, usually over a cup of tea.

A similar routine was followed in the afternoon. I had few visits to do. It was a joy to be taught by a man like Charles. In spite of it being a pretty dreary area, I found in him an immediate warmth and breadth of understanding, coupled with a remarkable level of academic knowledge for that time. And, of course, the variety of problems I was seeing was even broader than I had experienced over the previous six months. I had been right about anything coming through the doors of Casualty, but in general practice it was not anything – it was everything.

One day we finished earlier than expected. Charles went through our instructional routine with his usual thoroughness, and we were still ahead of time. At this stage it has to be said that his wife, Emily, was rather fierce. While very charming, as a retired operating theatre sister she liked things done her way – exactly as and when she ordained. Discipline was an essential part of her life. This morning Charles was in quietly mischievous mood.

'John, we seem to have done rather well this morning. If you have no further matters to raise, I think I shall go home early, stamp my foot and say to Emily, "What, lunch not ready?"'

I never did learn her response to that.

Quite apart from the greater variety of clinical material coming through the door of the little 'shop', the other marked change I found was that I was expected to make my own on-the-spot decisions as to what to do about each patient, without anybody looking over my shoulder. Of course, if I were stumped I could always seek help from Charles, but I rapidly found that I was managing quite well on my own – most of the time. And there was always the end-of-morning teaching session to look forward to.

Charles introduced me to the staff at a nearby children's hospital – just so that I could be known to them if I needed their help. He also introduced me to the local police station. The astonishing tranquillity of my start in the practice had to be broken by some sort of drama. One morning I saw a middle-aged lady with a nasty cough. I thought it might possibly be a bronchitis. I took Beth's history, making a few notes in her record, examined her chest carefully and advised as to the appropriate treatment for the bronchitis she certainly did have. I also wrote her the necessary prescription. I had not until then taken adequate note of the fact that she was accompanied by her aged mother. Or that it was the old lady who did all the talking. It was she who now intervened. There was another problem, her daughter also had pain in her knees. This was my first encounter with the 'while you are here, doctor' syndrome and it was by no means my last. I dutifully looked at the offending joints – they were not swollen, they were not red or hot, they were not tender and they moved through a perfectly acceptable range. They seemed pretty normal to me. So I said so.

It was only then that mother came up with the further information that the pain was not in the joints themselves, but in the lumpy bits below the knees – the tibial tuberosities. I had another look, this time at the right bits. Sure enough these were distinctly tender. Of course, I should have known that it was not her knees that were troubling her. I should not have needed telling. It was old Mrs Fernley who continued the dialogue – in a distinctly aggressive manner.

'Well, doctor, now you've seen it, what's the cause of that?'

I reassured her that there was nothing sinister to worry about and rather flippantly suggested too much kneeling as the background cause. This proved a distinctly unwise comment. Mrs Fernley leapt from her chair in absolute fury, demanding very loudly that she should see the 'proper doctor'. Charles was just letting his last patient out when this uproar erupted – and everyone in the waiting room must have wondered what was going on. He came in very quietly and took the pair of them off to his consulting room, leaving me to stew. Within a few minutes he had pacified them and sent them on their way. Before calling his next patient in, he came back to my room.

'Well, you seem to have caused something of a stir today, John.'

'But what on earth did I do to deserve that outburst?'

'Nothing, my dear fellow. Not really. I'm afraid your prime

fault was that you were quite right – they are a pair of religious fanatics. But you weren't to know that. It's called learning by experience. Keep at it.'

And then he had introduced me to my new patient and got on with his next one. I never discovered quite how he had so swiftly pacified the Fernleys. On reflection, I should have asked him more about that, as well as his wife's response to his early arrival for lunch.

I thought back to an incident during the war, when, as a junior signals officer, I was on loan to a Royal Artillery colonel for a week or so. He was quite a character. He greeted my arrival that first evening very fiercely. 'What the hell do you think you're going to do?'

'It all depends upon what it is you want, Sir.'

Perhaps that had not been the most diplomatic way I could have put it. We discussed his problem briskly. Then it was time for three of us to have supper together, Colonel Chapman, his regimental medical officer and me. Discovering that I had been a medical student in 'real life' the three of us talked into the night. I shall never forget the Colonel's final words.

'Remember only this – be he regimental medical officer, specialist or general practitioner, your doctor should be a man, and he may adorn his manhood with five years, ten years or a lifetime of study. It's time we all went to bed. There is a lot to do in the morning.'

A surprising insight for a gunner. But how right he was. My lifetime of study was still quite near its beginning.

The striking thing about this rather primitive practice was that so many patients were grateful for what help we could offer them. I found this particularly pleasant, and I felt sure that it was the natural outcome of a good consultation – it seemed to be an automatic response to the doctors being open and friendly towards their patients. Mutual respect seemed to me to be at the very core of things. I had certainly made the right decision in coming to Paddington for my initiation into general practice.

After three or four months, Charles asked me what sort of practice I thought I would like to end up in. I told him that I thought rural practice would suit me best, as I already had a love for the countryside and for country people. He warned me that this might involve even greater commitments, including dispensing, and delivering many young mothers at home. He went on to suggest that I should now start looking for an opening, so that I would not be left in limbo when I had finished my six-month term with him. This was very generous of him and I took his advice.

Within a month or so, after having a look at a few possibilities in Lincolnshire, Essex and South Wales, I really thought I had found my niche in rural practice in what used to be Huntingdonshire (until the clever politicians abolished the county). Even as an assistant, with a view to partnership, I would start at about two and a half times my gross pay in Casualty. And on top of that there was a small car allowance, because of the considerable amount of travel necessary for two doctors to cover thirty-seven villages and hamlets, night and day. It seemed pretty good. Charles immediately accepted that this sounded the right sort of practice for me, and insisted that I leave him early, as my prospective boss was in urgent need of someone as soon as possible. I spent a further two weeks with Charles – full of interest and as near tranquillity as can be reasonably expected in general practice. I owe a great debt of gratitude to Charles.

4

Real Work

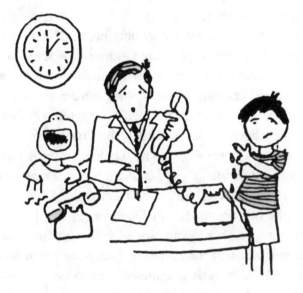

My new boss was a serious Scot, born and bred in Glasgow where he had qualified as a doctor after first taking a degree in biochemistry. Robert had been in my newly adopted county for only about five years, having settled there on coming out of the Royal Army Medical Corps at the end of the war. He had spent his first year as an assistant with a view to partnership, after which he became a partner with the ageing doctor, Jacob. The old man had declared that he would retire if the new fangled NHS came into being, but when this happened in 1948, he did not. This bred a rather unhappy atmosphere, which I imagine did nothing to make dealing with patients any easier – and none of them seemed to the Glasgow laddie to speak proper English, either. These East Anglian vowels were just not right to a Scot.

Before very long old Jacob finally retired, on completing a remarkable fifty-two years in the practice. Not only did he have a degree in public health, he had the distinction of having a second higher degree, his thesis for his Cambridge MD having been on the subject of anaemia in pregnancy – this in 1901, before anyone had heard of ante-natal care. To the astonishment of his pregnant patients, he had descended upon them at home and demanded that he take blood. He had made his own haemoglobin estimations in his private laboratory in an attic at his lovely old home. His patients thought it very odd that he should be visiting them when there was nothing wrong – and taking blood was most unnatural. Old Jacob had also written a book on archaeology.

When the old doctor did finally retire, Robert had hurriedly brought in a young man who proved to be quite unsuited to the job. The new assistant had lasted six months, before he had finally cast him out. With such a scattered area to cover, Robert was desperate to find a replacement, and determined that he would not make the same mistake twice. Perhaps in part because I had seen wartime military service, Robert had picked me for interview out of over forty applicants. I had dashed up from London and spent a challenging Sunday afternoon with him. In the midst of our discussion, he had had an urgent call from a village some miles away. We had gone together, and I had been able to take a rather closer look at the countryside as we drove.

Going west from the practice centre, we were in the 'hilly' part East Anglia – some of it over one hundred and fifty feet above sea level. Mostly it was arable land, with a considerable acreage under grass and numerous copses, reminiscent of Constable watercolours. I had yet to see the flat side – the endless stretch of featureless fenland to our east, with its enormous skies. Robert's call had been to an elderly lady with a painful cough. He had not invited me to see her with him, as I was not yet a member of the practice, but we had discussed her case all the way home. I was greatly impressed by the way he told her story. A quiet and very reserved man, he had taken a meticulous history and had clearly been thorough in his examination. His deductions seemed sound, and he had been able to do the necessary dispensing from the car, before leaving the patient. He had also given her a definite date for his next visit – the next day. This seemed to me to be real medicine.

I decided on the way back to his house that I wanted to work with this man. Over a cup of tea Robert had laid out his terms.

'I think we can work together very happily. As you can see, with the area to cover in this practice, I need someone very quickly. My offer is this. You will start as an assistant with a view to partnership at a salary of nine hundred pounds per annum – plus two hundred pounds as a car allowance. This will last one year. After this you will become a partner, at a one third share, increasing in stages to equality over ten years. If you can get released from your current commitment within three weeks, the job is yours.'

So, thanks to the very helpful Charles, here I was, just two weeks later, knocking on Robert's door on Sunday afternoon – for the second time. He had arranged digs for me with an elderly spinster named Gwen, a few miles from his house. I was to bring up the family as soon as we had agreed that we could work together. Robert's experience with his previous assistant had made him very cautious. He introduced me to my new landlady, I dropped off my bags, and then we went to 'my' surgery – a small cottage on the High Street of the biggest of 'our' thirty-seven villages. Here he gave me a map, showed me something of the geography of the practice and taught me the elements of dispensing – in about half an hour. The nearest pharmacy was ten miles away. It was quite a challenge.

Then he gave me the keys to the surgery and went home, telling me that I should start at nine the next morning and take local instructions from my landlady. Patients requiring visits would telephone her, and at the end of the morning surgery I should return to her house, when she would give me a list of visits to do, together with topographical and probably social instructions. On returning to Gwen that first Sunday evening I was given an excellent supper, by which time I was ready for bed. I reported to Mary that I was safe and sound and told her I would ring her again the next day. I slept like a log.

When I arrived at the surgery just before nine the following morning, there were already two patients waiting for me. They had chosen to stay outside, although the door was unlocked and Bertha Reynolds, the cleaner, was busy within. More of her later. My first patient was a tired-looking old man, the second a robust lady of forty or so, wearing baggy trousers and Wellington boots and armed with a hefty crook. After dealing with the old man's simple request for a repeat prescription (my first unsupervised filling of a bottle), Maud confronted me. I invited her to sit down.

'I won't sit down, doctor. I just need a bottle of cough stuff for a little girl.'

Maud was not best pleased when I said I would like to see the child first. She wanted to get back to work as a farm labourer.

Reluctantly she agreed that I should look in during the afternoon, giving me directions as to how to find the cottage, just outside one of the remoter hamlets on my 'beat', which lay way down in the fenland to the east. She stumped off looking daggers at me. I forget what I saw during the rest of that first surgery session. Consulting Gwen at the end of it, I got my marching orders and set off on the cross between a route march and a safari that was to characterise my mornings for many years to come.

This was to include my first experience of a 'call-house' – a cottage in one of the outlying villages where patients could see the doctor on five mornings a week and where they could also leave requests for repeat medicines or visits. The front room was available as a makeshift consulting room, while anyone else waited with Mrs White in the kitchen. A cupboard in the living room housed a supply of basic drugs, bottles, corks, labels and pill-boxes. As I was soon to learn, I had to remember to take spare supplies with me for any necessary topping up of stocks. In this sort of area, where few patients had transport of their own and there were no buses, I was to find that this rather primitive system worked pretty well. On this my first day I went to back to Gwen for lunch after two or three more stops by the way.

The western part of the area was very pleasant. Apart from the gently rolling hills, and the patchwork of grassland, crops and woodland I had noticed on my first visit to the practice, there was a medley of pretty little villages, their churches almost always with the fenestrated spires typical of the neighbourhood. It was indeed a green and pleasant land. And the people I met all seemed very down-to-earth and friendly.

After lunch it was time to find my way down the fen. This was a featureless countryside, with nothing to stop the biting east wind in two thousand miles from the Ural mountains. My directions had been adequate and I got to Maud's small cottage. It was rather gloomy and distinctly chilly. Little Margaret was making a horrid sound on coughing, and she was a nasty shade of blue. She was sick all right. Seriously so. I helped her take off her outer garments, only to run into unexpected trouble – she had been sewn into her vest and knickers for the winter. I next discovered that under the vest she was liberally smeared with what I learned was goose grease. This must have been a fen practice going back generations. To my horror, when I finally got down to skin I found that she had a full-blown lobar pneumonia. Happily, the village sported a phone box, only a few hundred yards away. Only minutes later I had spoken to the local hospital and ordered an ambulance, returning to the cottage to find little Margaret really very groggy. Maud thought I was making an awful fuss.

'I don't want my little girl to go to 'ospital, doctor. All she needs is a bottle of cough stuff.'

True, the hospital was nearly ten miles away from home, and Maud had no means of getting there to see her little girl – but I still did not agree. Thank goodness I put my foot down. In the event, Margaret recovered after nearly two weeks in hospital, and I never asked her mother whether the goose grease had been re-applied on her return home. But what an introduction to rural practice!

I made a few more visits before I settled down to the evening surgery. By the end of my first day I had seen a rare mix of patients, young and old, with life-threatening and relatively trivial complaints. And only Maud seemed displeased. Before leaving the surgery I filled up the depleted stock bottles for the morrow – the cough mixture, the upset stomach mixture and the one for

34

diarrhoea. Each contained about three litres of double-strength medicine, to be watered down for each patient. The recipes had been written down for me by Robert. They sounded truly nineteenth century – but they were all in the pocket pharmacopoeia I had bought before leaving Paddington.

At last I returned to my digs. Gwen wanted to hear what sort of day I had had, and she was pretty free with her comments on the people I had seen. She seemed to have an awful lot of information about an awful lot of people. I was not so sure that was a really good thing, but there was little I could do about it for the moment After my supper I had a call from Robert.

'Well, what sort of day have ye had? D'ye think ye'll survive?'

I reassured him as to the likelihood of my surviving. We then discussed a number of patients I had seen, and Robert reassured me that Maud only looked sulky – she was really quite a good egg, though perhaps a bit too self-reliant. He knew about the goose grease, too. And he was also well aware of the dangers inherent in Gwen having so broad an insight into other people's affairs. But there was little we could do about this for the time being.

'Did Maud leave a lot of mud in the surgery? I bet she was wearing her great boots. They say she goes to bed in them.'
I was reminded of the odd couplet I had come across many years before. Was it one of Hilaire Belloc's gems?

> The women of Nîmes are broad in the beam,
> But the men of St. Neots go to bed in their boots.

'When we have made up our minds about you staying here, we will get your family down and your wife can be the unpaid telephonist/receptionist for your beat, just like Nora is for mine. For now, I think I should let you get to bed. Good night, John.'

What a start to my rural life. At the end of the day, what mattered most to me was that this promised to be the right choice. I rang Mary to report on my first day's country practice. She sounded such a long way away. I needed a firm decision very soon, so that I could have her with me once more. Again I slept like a log – with no night calls, either.

Everything was so exciting, the time rushed past. Each day I was more certain that this was the practice for me, and Robert had pretty similar ideas, too. It was not long before we had agreed about that, although I would still not become a partner until the end of my first year in the practice. Few people would accept such terms today – but I had the security I needed, that was what mattered most. I started looking for somewhere to house Mary and the children. For a start I settled on renting half an old rectory, not two miles from the practice centre, and the family arrived in a snow storm. Our landlord was a delightful farmer, who lived in the other half of the house. Henry could not have been more helpful to the newcomers. Our water supply was from our own well, and we had an enormous pump in the kitchen, driven by an old Petter engine. I still have little idea how it worked, but it served us well, chugging away very effectively even if it was a bit noisy and smelly. So I was able to abandon Gwen in more ways than one, as I now had my very own telephonist/receptionist – like Nora, unpaid.

It was only days before Mary had an evening call from a strange voice from an outlying hamlet, while I was already out seeing a lad with whooping cough. Joan was asking if the doctor would call to see her brother. Mary enquired what was the problem.

'Well, Mum, I think 'e's got ole moanyer.'

Mary was really puzzled by this response – and, as Robert had, she found the East Anglian vowels very strange. Not unreasonably she asked for a bit more detail.

'I think 'e's got ole moanyer. You see, Mum, last year 'e had new moanyer, and e's jest the same this time – 'e's coughing like an old 'orse and 'e's got pain in 'is chest.'

Mary took directions from her caller as to how to find the place, and waited for me to get home. I got out of the car only long enough to learn where to go next. It was bitterly cold when I reached Ted's cottage. Yes, Joan had been right. Her brother had pneumonia – my second case in a few weeks. Ted was in pretty poor shape, and I went up to the village kiosk to phone the hospital, just as I had in the case of poor little greasy Margaret, way down the fen. And again I phoned the ambulance service. I had to have him admitted, as there was no way he could be adequately cared for where he was. Then I went back to prepare Ted and his wife for the journey to hospital and started on my way home. It had been a long day.

At this time I was driving a little Fiat Topolino. It had a tiny 500cc engine, but it was enough for me to get around the practice pretty cheaply. And that mattered – in spite of my recent increase in pay. On my way home I suffered more and more pain in my left big toe joint. By the time I arrived at the old rectory it was excruciating. Safely in the warm kitchen I struggled out of my shoe and sock only to find the joint grossly swollen, a vivid red in colour, and very tender to touch. Oh, Lord, what a bore, I must have gout. I could do without that! It was Mary who put me right.

'You old silly! It's a chilblain. Haven't you had one before? I had dozens of them when I was in my teens. They're horrid.'

Yes, the Topolino's floor was very thin and very close to the ground. The rubber mat was also very thin. I had never before had a chilblain, and for that matter I have never had one since. But I certainly did not enjoy this second brief experience of being a patient – the first being when I had driven myself (alone) seventy-four miles in a three-ton truck to have my appendix removed in the British General Hospital in Poona. The only other occasion had been my encounter with the professor of dentistry, during my first few weeks as a doctor. One thing was sure – it was certainly preferable to be the doctor rather than the patient.

The matter of feet reminds me of a story Robert told me about his wartime service as a regimental medical officer. He saw rather too many cases of foot rot. Demanding personal hygiene and meticulous sock washing did little to reduce the incidence of recurrences. Robert hit upon the perfectly reasonable idea that the culture medium had to be in the boot. So he changed tactics – he filled the men's boots with a concentrated solution of formaldehyde overnight. This killed off the causative organism rapidly, with complete success and Robert never saw a recurrence – but the troops didn't half stink.

It was only two or three weeks later that Mary had another call from Joan. She was very apologetic, telling Mary that her brother was home and doing well, but that her sister-in-law, Betty, had a bad pain in her tummy. To be on the safe side, Mary asked whether she might be pregnant. She was assured that this was not the case – but the pains were something awful. Once more I was already out, but Mary assured Joan that I would come as quickly as possible. As soon as I got home I was told to turn round and go to see the suffering Betty pretty smartly. Off I went, without checking whether I might need to take anything else with me – dreading another cold drive in my little car. Not another chilblain, please. Winter was by no means over.

The cottage was almost as cold as the car. At least I did not have to search for it – I knew where it was all right. There was no electricity, and the sole light in the place was from a single Petromax pressure lamp. The place was not only cold and gloomy, it was in a complete shambles. It was a real tip. Bearing the lamp with him, Ted led me through a jumble of furniture in the kitchen/living room into the bedroom at the back, where I found Betty well into the second stage of labour. This was no time for discussing Joan's assurance that Betty was not pregnant. In spite of the fact that he had only been home from hospital a few days, I dispatched Ted to the freezing telephone kiosk down the lane to summon the midwife. I asked him to be sure to tell her that I had not got my midwifery gear with me. I very much hoped I would not need it.

To the muted roar of the lamp, I delivered the baby in no time. It was Betty's first baby, but thank heavens it was a very easy birth. But what could I do with the wretched infant? There was nothing prepared for its arrival, there was no midwife present, and Ted had yet to return from the telephone kiosk. There was only one thing to do. I pulled out one drawer from the very scruffy chest of drawers. Dumping its contents unceremoniously onto the kitchen table I pulled the rather grubby eiderdown off the new mother and put a very healthy-looking child into its makeshift cot. It was only then that Ted returned, saying the midwife was on her way. Shaking his head in disbelief he said, 'I can't understand it, doctor. We'd no idea she were 'avin' a baby.'

I halted his explanation, suggesting that he find something to cover up his rather chilly wife. The midwife duly arrived, and I admit that I departed the scene as soon as I decently could. Never again did I drive anywhere without ensuring my midwifery bag was in the car, as well as my routine day-to-day bag and my emergency bag – and a spare can of petrol and a tow-rope for good measure. In fact, I only used the tow-rope to pull other motorists out of snow-drifts, and not with the Topolino, but that is another story.

In those first few weeks I was indeed glad that I had served under the great obstetrician who had made us all laugh so much about his colleague's flies. Of the first six babies I delivered at home, Betty's was the only normal case. The other five all involved some sort of abnormality. The most memorable of these was Alice's – another first baby. Alice was attended by the midwife who had delivered her, twenty-odd years before. This good lady did not seem to approve of my inexperience, and she kept a very watchful eye on this young 'country bumpkin' doctor.

The baby's head appeared a nasty shade of blue. The umbilical cord must be round its neck. I quickly had a look for this. It was true. I took off a loop. The colour of the infant's head did not improve at all. Yes, on looking again, I found the cord was still round the neck. I took off a second loop. Again, no improvement. In a very short time I had taken off no fewer than six loops, and the baby's colour responded at last. I had never heard of a cord being six times round an infant's neck. Nor had I imagined there could be a cord almost five feet long. Yes, I measured it later! All then went well, and I even had a subdued word of approval from the steely-eyed midwife. Alice and her delightful husband became very good friends of ours. And in the twenty five years I remained in general practice, I never lost a single mother or baby in home confinements.

Alice's husband, Gerald, was a great practical joker. Not many weeks later Mary answered the phone.

'Is that the doctor's? It's Mr Gotobed 'ere. I'd like 'im to call next time e's this way.'

Mary was not to be fooled. 'Don't try that one on, Gerald. You haven't fooled me, you chump.'

A very surprised Mr Gotobed then had to persuade Mary that he really existed, and that he did want the doctor to call. In fact Gotobed was not an uncommon name in that part of the world.

Bert was a funny old man. He came to see me one day, complaining of problems with his waterworks. This demanded an appropriate examination. I told him what I was going to do, got him onto the couch, lying on his side with his knees pulled up and I put on a rubber finger stall. Before I could get any further, he suddenly rolled onto his back, nearly tumbling off the couch, and grabbed my wrist – just like the lady in the 'ring clinic' in my first week as a doctor.

'Doctor, ought I to take my teeth out?'

I reassured Bert that this would not be necessary. I sincerely hoped he had no teeth the end I was about to investigate. I kept my laughter until after he had gone.

Sandra was seventeen. Sweet seventeen would not be the description that first leaped to mind. She was about the same height as I was. While I weighed nine stone five pounds, she topped me by something like three and a half stone. She was quite revoltingly fat. At least she acknowledged that she was overweight, but she was not much good at dealing with the problem. Someone had urged her to seek my advice. I tried to get her to understand that her weight gain was due to taking in more than she needed for the way she was made and for her way of life, but it was an uphill struggle. I wrote her out a simple diet sheet (which I used, slightly modified, very successfully for many years after this) but to no avail. She lost not a pound in several weeks, although she swore blind that she was doing what I had told her. After some time I got a bit impatient.

'Sandra, it's quite obvious that you are cheating. You are not doing as I say. You are wasting your time as well as mine. If you can't play ball with me, please go away.'

Poor Sandra burst into tears. I felt awful. But what could I do, if she was not going to cooperate? Later that day Helen my district nurse called in to see me.

'What have you been doing to our Sandra? She's dreadfully upset by you telling her to go away. Would you like to know what she's doing wrong?'

I spluttered something about her non-cooperation and the resulting waste of time, adding that she just could not be telling me the truth, and that I had better things to do.

'You're wrong there, doctor. You have been telling her about how much not to eat, and she has been doing just what you said. The problem is that she did not understand that fluids were included in the restriction. The silly girl still drinks two pints of sickly sweet lemonade every day.'

I modified my simple diet sheet that day. Fluids counted as much as did solids. Only then was it sound advice for the patient to follow my home-made diet sheet. A year or two later I showed it to a distinguished professor who was a world authority on nutrition, telling him that I thought counting calories was useless for most people and only increased the chance of the patient giving up. His response was encouraging.

'I've spent a long time thinking about these matters. I can't fault your approach.'

So, here it is.

NO
Chocolate or sweets
Sweet cakes or pastries
Sugar in tea or coffee
Nibbling between meals

EAT your normal diet

BUT take three quarters of your usual helping of everything else (except for a whole boiled egg!)

You should lose three to four pounds a week.
If you do not, you must be
ch**EAT**ing

I spoke to Sandra after the nurse's visit, apologising for upsetting her. Thanks to Helen, she made excellent progress after this.

Another occasion when misunderstanding occurred was in the case of Mrs Rialto. She was the wife of one of the quite numerous Italian ex-prisoners of war who had settled in the neighbourhood. While most of the ex-POWs lived in wartime Nissen huts, the Italian men worked largely on farms, learning enough English to cope with the boss and the beasts. They lived mostly in isolated farm cottages, where the women folk had little communication with the outside world and learned little English. The College of General Practitioners had recently issued a series of four-page leaflets for the use of its members, giving a number of medical terms in several languages. I had bought those in German, Polish, Italian and French. They cost one shilling each. Mrs Rialto came into my consulting room with a small child on her arm. I reached for my Italian 'idiot's guide to medical consultations' and did my best. It must have sounded all right, as Mrs Rialto obviously assumed that I could speak Italian and gabbled away at a great rate. I was lost. She eventually realised this.

'Uno momento, dottore.'

With this she scuttled back into the waiting room, where she had a quick discussion with her next-door neighbour, who had brought her along to see me. Mrs Church was a true daughter of the fen, with little schooling but a heart of gold. She had much in common with the booted Maud of my first day in the practice. She rapidly solved the linguistic problem, and Mrs Rialto came back into my room all smiles.

'Oh, dottore, bambino no shit verra good.'

The precious leaflets told one what to say for a start, but gave no indication as to what one might get in response. I tore up all four.

There was another occasion when communication was difficult – for a very different reason. It was a sad moment. Jill was the wife of a very pleasant schoolmaster. She was a highly intelligent woman, even if she did bang on rather. And she often seemed to talk in riddles. On this occasion she had a very serious vascular accident at home, and I saw her very soon afterwards. I realised that she must be admitted to hospital with all speed. She was very seriously ill and extremely distressed. There was no time to go off to a public telephone box. The only alternative was to telephone the local hospital in her presence, but the houseman I spoke to was rather uncooperative. I found it immensely difficult to describe to him the urgency of having her admitted, without upsetting her even more. It was with some relief that I finally managed to persuade him to admit her. But what a waste of time. And what potential for disaster.

On the subject of telephones, you will not be surprised to learn that I had a phone installed in the surgery the day after Mary had joined me. But there is another telephone tale to tell, which does not reflect a patient of mine directly, but which I have laughed about for a very long time. It was some years later, after Robert had retired early, that I brought a partner into the practice. Maurice was a first-class doctor, if a trifle outspoken at times. He also had a wicked sense of humour and was a devout churchgoer. He dutifully took his four-year-old son to church one Sunday. William sat very quietly for most of the service. What a well-behaved little boy. But the sound of the communion bell was too much for him. His small voice rang shrilly through the church.

'Bloody phone.'

Soon after my difficulties with phoning the hospital in Jill's presence, I persuaded my bank manager to provide funds to build a new surgery. (I will have more to say about this in a later chapter.) The previous year I had won a postgraduate prize for a paper with the dreadful title 'The Organisation and Administration of a General Practice, including the design of practice premises and the equipment required'. The preliminary work had been done – now I would put it into practice.

The aforementioned undergraduate prize had had another aspect which was not totally pleasing. The presentation was made in the Great Hall of British Medical Association House, by none other than the President himself. It was part of a substantial celebratory meeting. A variety of prizewinners were assembled in the narrow space between the side of the hall and the great platform, each being summoned in turn to the stage, leaving by similar steps on the other side. When my turn came, I dashed up the five or six steps in great style, tripped at the top step and landed in a most undignified heap at the feet of the President. I went down the other side rather more cautiously.

The new building was a wonderful escape from my dingy cottage. It was specifically planned to make life easy for everybody. With no ancillary staff, it was planned to offer an obvious

45

route in and out – the patients just could not go the wrong way. They entered a small lobby to find three doors. The one on the right was labelled 'Waiting Room', opposite that was the WC, while the third, opposite the front door, was firmly labelled 'Private'. This last was, of course, the way out of my consulting room, so that patients did not need to go back to the waiting room unless they wished to. The other door in the waiting room was into my consulting room. So no receptionist was needed, as I invited patients in through one door and ushered them out through the other. They just could not get lost.

To save on cleaning, I had the floors tiled with a brand called Accotile. One morning I arrived a little early, to find an unknown patient chatting with the cleaner. Admiring the new premises, she asked what the tiles were. Bertha Reynolds thought for a moment.

'I think they're those acolytes.'

Dear Bertha, she was a marvellous ally. She had lost her husband many years before in a railway accident and she had lost her submariner son during the war. Her daughter lived in the village. So she escaped her sorrows by throwing herself into all sorts of activities. Not only did she clean the surgery, she rang the church bell and polished the brasses, she did teas for the British Legion and the Women's Institute, and she did the laying out for anyone who died in the village or nearby. She was never sick until she had a stroke at the age of almost eighty. Surviving this, she reluctantly agreed to stop her other pursuits. But she insisted on returning to work in the surgery. I thought I knew why she felt she needed to go on with that.

'Mrs Reynolds, why are you so keen on staying on in the surgery?'

Bertha smiled broadly. 'The old doctor served fifty-two years in the practice, didn't he – so I'm going to.'

'That you will have done this year, won't you? I don't suppose I shall match that.'

Yes, she beat the old doctor. Bertha was an absolute treasure. I missed her sadly when she eventually gave up work.

Firmly esconced in my little palace, using a small tape recorder to talk to myself in the car between visits, it was my initial custom to type letters myself at the end of the day. I really could have done with some part-time help, but I admit to putting it off. The last person in the waiting room one morning was a neat little lady with a rather delightful smile. I did not recognise her.

'Do sit down. What can I do to help you?'

'I'm not ill, doctor. My name is Beverley Grant – my husband and I have only very recently moved into the village. I have brought our cards along, but I do hope you will be able to help in another matter. As the local doctor, you must know an awful lot of people around here. I just wondered whether you knew of anyone who needed a part-time secretary?'

'Stay there, Mrs Grant. I do indeed. The first on the list is me.'

I set out on my morning visits in very good cheer. Beverley Grant had a job – I had a part-time secretary. It was ages before she admitted to me that she had intended just that to happen. Crafty thing, she really had manipulated me. She was wonderful.

There was no end to the variety in the practice. On one of my 'safaris' round the outlying villages, I saw an elderly widow with a very odd-looking knob on the end of her nose. I was almost sure it was malignant. While I always tried to be honest with patients, I needed to be sure. She asked me what she should do about it.

'Mrs Burdett, you look just like a rhinoceros. I think we had better have that off – pretty smartly.'

Happily she was not at all offended by my flippancy – indeed she laughed aloud at it. At that particular moment, for that particular patient with her potential problem, it was an excellent expression to use. I managed to get her brought down to the new surgery two days later, where I removed the offending growth. I was delighted to be able to make use of the plastic surgery skills learned in my first few weeks after qualification. I sent the specimen to the laboratory, where it was reported to be a 'proper' skin cancer. Was I glad I had got on with the job so quickly! In a week or so she had a scarcely visible scar, and she lived for a good number of years with no suggestion of recurrence. Delighted with the result, she never questioned me as to what the lump was. So I never volunteered the diagnosis.

She was almost embarrassingly grateful. After this, every year, just before Christmas and Easter, I would receive a note from her, the same wording each time.

'Dear doctor, when you are next in the village, please would you call. I have a few things for you to collect. And when you come, would you please bring some "lumbagoa tablets" for brother Alfred?'

Alfred was her bachelor brother, who kept a highly productive allotment just down the hill from the cottage they shared. They had a substantial chicken run in their garden. Each Christmas I would collect a score of enormous eggs (never a paltry dozen), three sticks of Brussels sprouts and some chocolates for the children. Each Easter there would be another score of eggs, a big box of lovely waxy potatoes and some Easter eggs. This sort of thing made the slog of practice so very worth while.

5

More of the Same Medicine

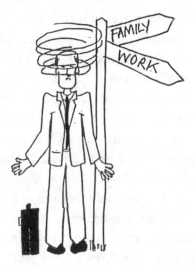

Perhaps one of the most rewarding things about country practice is its unlimited variety. In the early days I had thought that Casualty was the ultimate in unpredictability. In a few very educative months, Paddington taught me that I was wrong. Now I knew very much better. One of the delights I 'inherited' from Robert in my early days here was the story of Albert – a chronic schizophrenic man who lived not very far from Ted and his 'old moanyer', not to mention the non-pregnant Betty with the rather cold baby. A bachelor, Albert lived alone in one of a remote cluster of three cottages, happily with a very helpful couple next door. I never met the occupants of the third house in twenty-five years in the practice. Albert worked very happily as a farm labourer, except for his occasional 'turns'. When these came on, his good neighbours would very properly ring for help. They had their own telephone – the only one in the tiny hamlet.

In those days getting a mentally deranged patient into hospital was quite a palaver. The doctor had to arrange a meeting between himself, the 'duly authorised officer', a magistrate and the patient. The magistrate needed to sign the form of committal before the patient could be taken proper care of. Only then could the duly authorised officer take the patient to hospital. Somehow such emergencies always seemed to occur at weekends, when the doctor was almost certainly doing two people's work. This time was no exception. Not only was Robert on call for two doctors over the weekend, the 'duly authorised officer' was very busy gardening, and he was most reluctant to be involved. However, Robert persuaded him that his attendance was necessary. The next difficulty was finding a magistrate. At last Robert pinned one down – an excellent pork butcher from the nearby town. The meeting was arranged for three o'clock, and they were at last all four assembled around Albert's kitchen table.

Just as I had later found in the case of Jill's admission to hospital, Robert had some difficulty in presenting the case for commitment in Albert's presence, as he was afraid he might further upset the patient's very real instability. Though he knew Albert of old, the duly authorised officer was not at all supportive. He just wanted to get back to his garden. Unconvinced by Robert, the magistrate was in no mood to help either. After a while the worthy butcher decided that they were getting nowhere – he declared that he would conduct proceedings himself. He asked Albert a few questions, which he answered perfectly well. Yes, it was Saturday, Queen Victoria had been dead for a number of years, Albert's name was Albert, he was unmarried and this was his home. That somewhat cursory questioning seemed to satisfy the magistrate far better than Robert's wary description of a case of chronic schizophrenia.

'Doctor, you've heard the patient's answers to my questions. He's got every one of 'em right. I'm afraid I just can't sign this form.'

Robert was near to despair. Any further discussion could easily provoke a disaster. He just did not know what to say next. Mercifully for Robert, Albert himself came to the rescue. He got up from his chair rather ponderously, slowly shuffled round the corner of the kitchen table, and then suddenly stooped down and bit the magistrate's left ear. Never was a committal form signed so quickly! The duly authorised officer was galvanised into action, and moments later he and Albert were on their way to hospital, Albert clearly sensing the security this offered him. After all, he had been there before – more than once. This left Robert to stitch the bleeding magistrate's ear. While he attended to his new patient, he did just wonder what was the sense in requiring a pork butcher to make overriding decisions about complex psychological matters. What a daft arrangement. It could only have been a politician who though that one up .

Not very long after I heard this tale I experienced for myself another episode in relation to schizophrenia. It was Robert's weekend off duty. James was a known sufferer, with whom I had had nothing to do, as he lived in Robert's part of the practice area. But I was glad that I did know something of his case, if only by hearsay. He lived with his parents in a very remote bungalow in the middle of a beech wood, two or three miles away. Again inevitably on a Saturday afternoon he suffered sudden deterioration, and I was sent for. His parents were said to have fled, and were sheltering in a friend's house in the nearby village. I decided to see them first. James had beaten up his old father, cracking two ribs. The old man was, of course, pretty badly shaken and James's mother, who was stone deaf, was terrified. There was little I could do for mum, other than to reassure her that she was now safe. I quickly patched up dad and gave him some painkillers from the car, before going to the house in the woods.

Letting myself in, I found James standing at the far end of the corridor mute and motionless, one arm raised like a Greek statue. He was truly in the catatonic phase. I needed appropriate help. When I rang him, the 'duly authorised officer' – not the same one as had been involved with Albert – was very reluctant to come out. When he did come he was totally unhelpful, saying that James was doing nobody any harm standing in the passage. Thank goodness, due to a change in the law, I did not need to bother the pork butcher. He might not have been too keen on the idea, anyway. All I could do was to demand that the reluctant expert meet me at Robert's surgery. I had to get the Medical Director of the nearby mental hospital to speak to him on the telephone, before he would take any action. He was told very firmly that James must be brought into hospital without further delay. He was. I went back to two people's work.

Ernie was quite a prosperous old farmer who had come to the area as a small boy from Yorkshire, driving a herd of cattle all the way along the grassy drove roads that had been laid out in the Middle Ages. Over the years he had become one of the locals. He was a delightful chap, full of fun. He was deeply interested in his adopted community, and he had long served on the Rural District Council. With rather similar ideas about one's adopted community, I had been elected to the RDC a short while earlier, which I found most interesting, although it was very difficult to find the time to do it properly. The meetings were little trouble, but it was almost impossible to find time to look into potential problems before attending a meeting, so that one was better informed. When I could, I used to pick Ernie up and drive him to meetings in the local town.

One day, as we drove to a meeting, I was pulling his leg about recent agitation by the National Farmworkers Union. Not surprisingly, they were seeking a better deal for their members, and I teased old Ernie mercilessly about his being ruined through having to pay his men a decent wage. I shall never forget his reply.

'I allus tell them the same – you can't 'ave it till I've got it.'

This gem I reported to the Chancellor of the Exchequer of the day, who happened to be our local MP. He was delighted to hear Ernie's comment and we agreed that he was quite right. And yes, he knew the family, though not the old man himself. Unfortunately, my report of Ernie's wisdom was too late for the budget speech.

One of the refreshing things for me about being a councillor was that I never once heard mention of party politics at meetings – we were gathered to do something useful for our native or adopted community. But I did not serve long as country practice just did not allow the time to do the job properly. So with great regret I abandoned it.

Death is an inevitable aspect of general practice. Sometimes a blessing, sometimes a tragedy, it is just part of the scene. Two such occasions linger with me still. Once I had set up home in the area, I had had little to do with Gwen, my original landlady. She was always busy, looking after her rather trying old mother for a number of years and being a pillar of the Methodist Chapel. She was never one to complain, and I do not recall ever having had to do anything for her as a patient. I had been pretty busy, too. Out of the blue I had an urgent call to see her. I knew it must be serious, and I dropped what I was doing and dashed round at top speed. Poor dear, she had had a massive stroke, and was only just conscious. She was obviously pleased to see me and before she died, only minutes after my arrival, she managed one slurred sentence.

'I'm so sorry to be such a nuisance, doctor.'

And then she was gone. I was so glad I had got there in time for her end.

Mollie was an even greater sadness for me. She had been my local district midwife when I first arrived on the scene. I had found her a bit fierce to start with, but I learned to appreciate her stalwart work as the years passed. She guided me through many a trying time, and she certainly contributed to my success in dealing with childbirth in the cottage – as previously reported, in twenty-five years I never lost a single mother or baby in childbirth. Not long after she retired she developed a peculiarly nasty cancer. There was no question as to what it was, and there was no way it could be cured. I knew it and she knew it. So palliative care in her own home was all that was left to us. Poor dear, it was not much fun for her and, in spite of my efforts to ease the pain and cheer her up, she suffered a great deal of distress. Her son lived far away, her daughter had a small baby to deal with. Inevitably Mollie slowly deteriorated. In the end she despaired.

'Doctor, I've had enough. Will you help me? Please.'

She was so quiet and dignified. There was no drama about her request. Neither was there any doubt as to what she was asking me to do. I was faced with a very difficult decision. I have never been in doubt as to what I should have done – in her best interest. Should not the anguish of the individual patient take precedence over the impersonal principles of the State, the Church and the medical profession?

One day Derek came to see me. He was a retiring sort of chap, still in his twenties, who had recently finished his National Service as a pilot in the RAF. Of course I should have known better, but I once more failed to appreciate the significance of a responsible adult being accompanied to the surgery by his mother – and mother doing most of the talking. Shades of Paddington High Street and the painful knees. No religious mania here, just a difference of opinion. When I made a tentative diagnosis, mother did not agree.

'Nonsense, doctor. Surely he can't have it again. He's had it twice before once at school and again in the RAF.'

Now it was my turn. I reckoned I knew better than this rather bossy lady.

'Nonsense, Mrs Pratt. Contracting the condition gives rise to permanent immunity. It can only occur once.'

That consultation took far too long. We could not agree at all. After some persuasion, I took some blood and sent it off for a repeat blood test and told the pair of them that I would look into the matter further. Derek's test came back positive – at least I was right in my diagnosis. So, after informing Derek of the definitive diagnosis and making an alteration to his medication, I wrote to the medical officer of his old school and to the RAF medical branch, seeking evidence with regard to the alleged previous attacks. Both replied that the results of their tests had been positive. To my astonishment and great delight both went further, to say that repeat tests six months later had proved negative. This was not at all what I had been taught. So I wrote to my old teaching hospital for advice. The end-result was that Professor Biggs and I wrote a short paper on the case, the first time in medical history that such a sequence had been reported. Sadly Derek – I suspect on mother's advice – declined to give blood for a follow-up test six months thereafter, which would have made the evidence that much stronger. This was my introduction to the writing of professional papers – there were a lot more to come.

I am reminded of an entertaining tale related to this story. At one time we had a delightful German au pair. Heidi became very much a part of the family, and indeed we visited her in Germany many years later, after she was married. Her sister had come over at the same time, and she was living with Derek's mother – very much in the kitchen. Mathilde's English was not nearly as good as Heidi's. Each morning the jovial local postman used the same greeting for the buxom Mathilde at the kitchen door.

''Ow are yer?'

Each day the poor girl's smiling reply was not entirely appropriate. Somehow she misunderstood the East Anglian vowel sounds. They were not at all like Hochdeutsch.

'Mathilde Grünbaum.'

It was Heidi who sorted her sister out in the end, but this odd exchange was to be repeated daily for a week before this happened. We all had a good laugh about it – at nobody's expense. I thought about Robert's difficulty with East Anglian vowel sounds when he came down from Glasgow. But I never learned what the postman made of Mathilde's responses to his daily greeting.

Mrs Ball was a bit of a know-all. She was a regular attender at meetings of the parent/teacher association at the village primary school. At one meeting Mary went to she was sitting in the row in front. Someone was giving a talk on pre-history – perhaps not the most suitable of topics for her rather primitive village audience. After some minutes Mrs Ball's immediate neighbour leaned towards her.

'What's a Dianasore, then?'

The reply came out loud and clear – loud enough to astonish the speaker and make her falter in her stride.

'I think it's a medieval animal.'

It is sometimes easy to be misunderstood. One day a rather grubby, fat, middle-aged lady appeared in the surgery, complaining of pain in her right shoulder. I invited her to sit down, while I took her history.

'Let's take a look then – just take a few things off, please.'

Before I finished writing her notes, I was interrupted by the telephone. I completed the record before getting up from my desk. The patient was lying flat on her back on the couch – stark naked. It was a distinctly disconcerting sight. I hurriedly suggested that she should put on a few things before I examined her shoulder. I think I did her some good after that – but I found it a horrifying experience. I certainly should have learned from that, but in fact I did something similar again, as you will learn later.

It is funny how one does not always understand what others expect one to understand. I had had a weekend off duty, with Maurice, Robert's successor, standing in for me. On Monday morning I went in early to look at any notes he might have left me. Two seemed perfectly straightforward, if a bit difficult to make out, as his writing was very poor. The third was to do with a pleasant, rather scatterbrained lass in the next village. I knew her quite well, and I was not entirely surprised that she should have found it necessary to call Maurice out. I struggled with the notes for quite a while. I had always felt strongly about writing things legibly – being able to read it is surely what writing is for. But I was defeated by the only bit I could read with ease. There it was, at the bottom of the sheet, in capitals – NAFC.

I rang Maurice to ask him what he had found wrong with the lass.

'Maurice, what on earth does NAFC mean?'

'Oh, John, don't you know?'

'Of course I don't know – otherwise I wouldn't be ringing you now, would I?'

'I thought everybody knew that one. Nutty as fruit cake.'

I certainly never forgot NAFC as a diagnosis – it summed up quite a lot in four letters. And there were times when it seemed most appropriate. No one would dare to write that today. The legal repercussions would probably be disastrous.

Driving a car was an important part of country practice – there were many miles to cover in a year. I got rid of my 'ice-box' Topolino pretty quickly. As my mileage was inevitably high, I thought it best to buy a modest car and to change it after about a year for something with less on the clock. It was the schoolmaster husband of the deceased Jill who pointed me in the right direction. As a sideline, with a colleague he ran a small business nearby, renovating and selling nothing but old Rolls Royces and Bentleys.

'John, you now drive like an angry Frenchman. With the Rolls Royce your whole style will change – you will drive with dignity.'

He introduced me to a charming twenty-two-year-old Rolls Royce. It seemed enormous, with a vast bonnet sticking out in front and great wide running boards on either side – and enormous wheels. I bought it for £500. It was an absolute joy. In spite of its engine capacity it was remarkably economical to run – twenty-two miles to the gallon – and all I bought for it in a year was two tyres. After putting twenty-five thousand miles on the clock, I turned that one in and received a second (lower mileage) one – with no financial transaction at all. In the end I had a series of six old Rolls Royces for my original £500. In spite of my adding a substantial mileage to each one, their escalation in capital value was sufficient for my good friend to allow me this joy – and I had no repair bills at all in six years. And yes, my style of driving was transformed from day one. I do so wish I had been able to keep one. Unhappily, I had nowhere to store it and anyhow at that time I could certainly not afford that sort of luxury. That £500 was needed for my next car.

Now and again I managed to escape from work for short periods – not a bad thing really. One such escape was afforded by Harold, a landowner patient of mine, who occasionally invited me to shoot with him and a couple of his tenant farmers. Four 'guns' would meet at the castle and then walk miles over grass and arable land, with game-keeper Eddie and his lovely golden Labrador. Nothing up-market about it, no great slaughter done, but a lovely relaxing day in the fresh air. And towards the end of the afternoon we would return to the stables to sort things out. Eddie would lay out the bag, while Harold would meticulously enter each item in his game book. He was very particular about writing everything down in an orderly manner.

On one of these lovely days there was a pretty strong wind blowing, and we were plodding through a field of fairly well-grown sugar beet near the London–Edinburgh railway line. Because of the wind, the birds were sitting pretty tight, and I nearly trod on a beautiful cock pheasant before it flew off the way we had come in a noisy flurry. Swinging round pretty smartly, I had to use both barrels, but I got the bird. Eddie's Labrador went streaking off to pick it up. It was then that we heard a great shouting from a little way off. There was a man shaking his fist and swearing at us, leaning on the balcony rail of the nearby signal box. Some spent shot had rattled his window pane. No harm was done, so we left him to it and went on our way.

Some time later we returned to the stables, a little weary but very happy. Here the ritual sorting and entering took place. Between us we had not done badly. When all was done each of us guests was given a brace of pheasant to take home to our wives – a sort of peace offering for having 'played' while they worked. But before this we enjoyed a memorable moment. Harold had something of a stutter. Writing up his game book, he turned to his faithful game-keeper and thanked him for his help, adding. 'I s-say, E-eddie, I d-don't think we n-need to e-enter the doctor's s-signal box.'

Will was an elderly man who had worked his whole life for the same small builder. This meant several miles' cycle ride to and from the yard each day. He was used to that. But he had the misfortune to be diabetic, and was liable to episodes of hypo-glycaemia from time to time. He usually coped with these tiresome attacks pretty well, always carrying a few lumps of sugar with him wherever he went. Well, not quite always. One day he was on his way home after a day's work, spinning down the last small hill to his village, when he felt distinctly groggy. Fishing in his pocket he found no sugar. His speed increased as he got further down the hill and he finally fell off his bike. Soon after this a neighbour came by in his car, picked Will up and took him home, before phoning the doctor.

By the time I got there Will had had his lump of sugar – if somewhat belatedly. He was feeling much better, though a trifle bruised and rather ashamed of himself for not having his sugar to hand. He described to me the actual place where he had landed. In fact, his neighbour had picked him up from a large heap of sugar beet – several tons of it – awaiting the truck to take it to the sugar beet factory.

'You're a right chump, Will. You only needed to have a gnaw at the beet, and you would have ridden home as usual.'

One rather unusual episode occurred before Robert retired. He was off duty when the local police telephoned him to ask his help over a drunk. Winnie was being very obstreperous outside a nearby pub. Robert told them he was not on call, so they asked him if he could suggest anything to quieten the lady. He had had a bad day. He felt he needed his short break from work.

'Have ye tried Horlicks?'

Perhaps this was not the most helpful of responses. In the end I had to go to the Royal Oak. What I found was dramatic. Two Irish labourers were lying unconscious on the pavement outside. A third man was sitting on a bench beside them, moaning and nursing his head. Winnie was swearing at all and sundry, lashing out at anyone who was rash enough to get within her reach. She needed sedating – very soon. Apart from two policemen, by this time no fewer than two ambulances had arrived – each with two attendants. I was not sure whether they had been called for her or for her victims. I tried argument, but I was immediately attacked. I found myself grappling with the good lady and rolling down the bank of a rather charming small stream. Shades of the Saturday night drunk in Casualty. At least I remained conscious and this time my specs were intact.

In the end, with the assistance of one of the ambulance drivers, I managed to restrain Winnie sufficiently to give her an injection.

Then we got her into one of the ambulances, still struggling pretty vigorously, where we wrapped her tightly in a blanket, and laid her on a stretcher. It was too soon for the injection to have taken its full effect, and it needed two ambulance men sitting on her to keep her there. With a certain lack of dignity she set off for hospital. Following in their wake, the fourth ambulance man took the three Irishmen. When I rang the hospital to warn them of what was in store for them, I was told that this was a matter for the police. The houseman declined to admit Winnie. I could only suggest that he decided about this on her arrival – she was already on her way. I went home, but not without having discovered that her brother had been a top-ranking boxer. I shudder to think how such an episode might be reacted to today – litigation in a big way.

Wally was a bit of a pain. He was not at all a pleasant man and had few friends – one soon found out why. As a farmer he was pretty competent, and he owned quite a lot of property in the region. He treated his wife very badly, and she ultimately 'abandoned ship' to live far away. He lived on alone, making himself a nuisance much of the time. In every activity he was mean and demanding. One of his traits was to always demand special treatment from his doctor. He made it sound so reasonable, and I was perhaps too gullible in not dealing with him more firmly from the start. Now and again he would seek to placate me by saying he would remember me in his will. He suffered a series of serious illnesses before finally giving up the ghost – to the frank delight of some. I had certainly had a great deal to do for him over some years. And I cannot say that I missed him sorely.

Months later I had a call from my solicitor. He was not a patient of mine, although I knew him quite well, as a member of a local debating society.

'In the case of Walter Firth, deceased. Don't think this is going to change your way of life ...'

Wally was as good as his word. The old devil had left me £20.

6

As if That Were Not Enough!

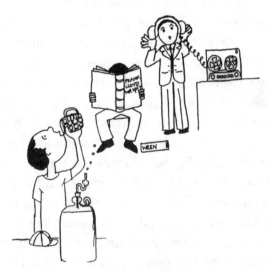

There was a time when I thought that general practice was a full-time job. On the face of it, this sounds a reasonable proposition. Derek's blood tests were not the only example of fresh ideas and fresh pursuits invading the time and space of the consulting room. Quite early on Ann came to seek my advice about adoption. She and her husband, Ben, had been hoping to have a baby for a couple of years, but with no result. They had heard that some people who adopted a child went on to have a baby of their own – was it true? Of course I had heard of this happening, but I had not actually come across it, and I had certainly not heard mention of it as an undergraduate. I had not thought very deeply about it either – let alone come up with any positive ideas. All I could do was to confirm that it did happen from time to time. Should they take steps towards adoption? I asked Ann and Ben to give me a few days to think about it. I needed to chew the cud. I would get back to them.

The more I thought, the more exciting the prospect seemed. Was it not true that all hollow organs could go into spasm on some sort of provocation? The gut could be very painful from this cause. The ureters could similarly be the origin of pain, if something caused them to go into spasm. Severe chest pain could arise from spasm of the coronary arteries. At least some of these could arise from emotional causes. The Fallopian tubes, connecting the ovaries to the uterus, were of similar structure – muscular tubes, with their own nerve supply. Why could they not go into spasm too? The fact that pain did not enter the scene did not seem to matter. Surely, in the event of tubal spasm, the ovum and the sperm would be kept apart – possibly long enough for the sperm to die. And why could such spasm not result from an emotional cause? More significant, why should one possible emotional cause not be a desperate desire to have a baby? Dreams – all dreams.

A day or so later I discussed my ideas with Ann and Ben. They accepted the possibility that I might have hit upon something. No more than that. I then suggested to them that we really should seek to prove the matter. They were definitely interested. My argument was that, if emotional tension lay at the root of their difficulty, then some sort of tranquilliser might prove effective in preventing the spasm resulting from that tension. There seemed to be two alternatives – for Ann to take either a slow-acting tranquilliser for a few days around the time of ovulation, or a rapid-acting tranquilliser half an hour before jumping into bed.

She and Ben were keen to give the idea a try. But I saw two problems. Which choice should I make? How could anyone accept that any success Ann and Ben might have was not just due to chance – or perhaps just to my having taken an interest in their problem? This required more thought.

The plan I formulated was really quite simple. We needed to have a number of couples take part in a small clinical trial. They had to be divided into four groups – two taking either one or other of the pills decided upon, two taking identical-looking dummy pills, none of the lasses involved knowing whether they were taking an active drug or a placebo. So far, so good. I next had to persuade two drug manufacturers to provide me (gratis) with the necessary drugs/dummy pills. This proved easy, and soon I had supplies in hand. There was never any suggestion of my being paid a fee, and I never even thought of it. I tried to involve my local obstetrician in the trial but, though she was quite intrigued by the idea, she was too busy to take on the extra work. I tried interesting GPs in the region. This proved much more encouraging – in a short time I had the trial under way. The choice of medication was determined by me, no one else knew which patient was taking an active drug or a placebo. Participating doctors had their supplies from me labelled by number only.

To her great delight, Ann was the first patient to participate in the trial. Ten months later, she produced a splendid infant, which I delivered in the local maternity hospital with equal delight. They were such a happy family. The problem with the trial, however, was that it took so long, and most of the doctors involved found themselves too busy to carry on with it. It took ages for me to get together thirty cases – six of them from my own practice. This was nowhere near sufficient to produce a statistically valid result.

Very disappointed, I abandoned the trial. But not before we had had six babies from the thirty mothers who had taken part – all of these taking an active drug, including Ann. Not one lass on either of the placebos became pregnant.

I suppose we may all be carried away with a particular enthusiasm. Even if it had proved nothing, my sub-fertility trial, though I cut it short, started something for me. I kept on having ideas. And I kept on wanting to pursue them. I suppose as a result of my having worked with wireless sets during the war, I had developed the ability to listen to small sounds while ignoring much louder ones. One day I was in the middle of my ante-natal clinic. On listening to one tummy I was astonished to hear what I was sure were abnormal foetal heart sounds. Yes, the 'proper' sounds were definitely accompanied by a very odd whooshing noise. I had certainly never heard of the possibility of discovering such a thing at this stage, but I was sure that it was there. When I told a colleague, he dismissed my idea as another of my dreams.

'Come off it, John. It's difficult enough being certain of an abnormal heart sound through the chest wall – and that after the patient has taken off coat, sweater, shirt and vest. Wrap it up in layers of abdominal muscle, gut, fluid, uterine muscle and more fluid, and you haven't a hope. It's nothing but wishful thinking. You old dreamer.'

I knew I was right. How could I convince people? Could I record it on tape? Why not? I already had a big old Grundig Reporter tape recorder. I bought an amplifier I could not really afford, and a rather sensitive microphone to go with it. I cadged a Jersey-sized liner for a milking machine from a local dairy farmer – to insulate the microphone a bit from room noises. I put everything together in great haste and looked for something to try it on. Our youngest child was being bottle fed. What a splendid coincidence. I started on him during a feed, so as to keep him at peace while I was doing my stuff. I recorded his heart sounds all right – and they were excellent. But there was something very odd about the recording – as well as the sounds I was expecting there was a very odd intermittent trilling – and it had no bearing on the heart's rhythm. It took a while for me to realise what this was. It was air bubbles entering the bottle between sucks. Perhaps that should have been obvious – at least I got the answer after a while.

I was only just in time. My patient went into labour only a day or so after I had got my new toys together and tested. I dashed to her house, arriving at the same moment as the midwife. All three of us knew what I wanted to do, the patient had had no qualms about being 'experimented on' and the midwife had agreed to do the actual delivery while I 'played'. It was a magic experience. Setting it all up in no time, I recorded the sounds I had heard in the clinic – if anything they were clearer now. I followed the infant's journey towards the outside world with great care. As soon as its chest appeared I transferred my microphone from mum's tummy to the child. There it was on tape. I had an unique recording – something to be treasured. This would quieten my critics. Here was real evidence. This was real research!

I started to pack up my toys, but the midwife motioned to me urgently. The wretched little babe had multiple deformities – as well as her serious heart condition she was obviously blind, she had one grossly abnormal arm and several extra toes. In my excitement over my ideas, I had not noticed any of these. This poor little child could never live an independent life. What a wretched end for my day, and how ghastly a sequel to my fascinating sub-fertility research. I felt terrible. Of course, the following year one of the big medical instrument makers produced a much better machine. Even so it was an interesting experience. And another first for me.

Perhaps it was not entirely a matter of chance that provoked my interest in depression. Looking back it is easy to see how it all started, but at the time I was far too riveted to my wonderful job to take much notice of myself. Of course my workload was heavy, but I did not mind that in the least – except that it meant that I had too little time with my family. Patients came first. I learned the hard way.

Lorna was seriously depressed. Not surprisingly she had a hideously complex background to her problems, and for a start I had found it difficult to help very much. She was clearly approaching suicide. One afternoon I was called to her cottage as a matter of urgency. Her neighbour was very worried about her. Lorna was beside herself with grief and despair. I do not remember quite what it was I said to her, but her expression suddenly changed and her awful jabbering stopped – as if by magic.

'My God, doctor, you've been there too.'

Of course, Lorna was right. Though previously not admitting it to myself, I was indeed quite seriously depressed. Happily I was able to help her much more after that dramatic exchange. And I began to understand myself a little better, too. And from that day on I added depression to the list of ailments I was actively looking for.

It also provoked me to further constructive thought on the subject. I slowly came to realise that everyone occupies a position on a sort of scale of depressibility – this is genetically determined. Apart from what I call 'genetic molesting', there is nothing one can do about it. The incidence of episodes of depression is always the result of the interplay between an often unidentified outside influence and this inherited factor. If you are at one end of the scale of depressibility your mother-in-law frowning may set off a depressive episode, while if you are at the other end of the scale it will take a major disaster.

If this is the case, the logical way to deal with such an episode must therefore be first to identify the outside cause, second to deal with this as best one can, and only third to treat the patient – if the problem still persists. This seemed to me the only rational approach. So anti-depressants must be best used in the short term to enable the patient to think straight and so to identify the outside factor. If it is possible to deal with this, the patient has no longer got a problem. If not, the patient needs assistance in learning to live with it. The common long-term use of anti-depressants seemed to me irrational. I pursued this approach over many years, with very rewarding results. It was certainly hard work. And it did little to help me.

Long before this I had had my interest in back pain stimulated by a series of odd incidents. I had seen numerous cases, mainly in farm workers doing pretty heavy work. Heaving and lugging bales and sacks, hedging and ditching, shoving large animals about, quite apart from any damage done by long periods sitting on a vibrating tractor seat going over bumpy ground, puts the farm worker at some risk of back problems. Brought up in the usual orthodox way, I had given these men painkillers and a sickness certificate and told them to have a few days in bed before seeing me again. Then I noticed something odd. Again and again I saw these chaps cycling off to work the following day. One after another I stopped them and asked what on earth they were up to. Their rather reticent reply was always the same.

'Oh doctor, I can't afford to be off work. I got a family.'

'But yesterday you were absolutely crippled. How the hell can you do your sort of work with a back like yours?'

The answer was the same, time and again. They had gone off to see the bone-setter in a neighbouring village, torn up their sickness certificates and stuffed their tablets in the back of a cupboard. Clearly I needed to learn something.

A sensible start seemed to be a visit to the bone-setter. I found him a very pleasant character, and we talked for quite a while. His training had been rudimentary – chiefly by the example of his wholly unqualified aunt, supplemented by a very odd collection of ideas as to how the human body worked. He showed me some techniques – for the life of me, I could not see what he was actually doing. What mattered was that he was enabling my failures to go back to work. There had to be some rationality behind it all. I did not really relish being made to look unnecessarily stupid or unhelpful.

There was only one man I could think of who might be able to help. I knew him slightly from my student days. Although many of his consultant colleagues poked fun at him, he had studied this enormous problem from a more or less orthodox medical point of view, and he had written a substantial book on the subject. So, apart from reading his book, I did a brief course with him, before trying out a few tentative techniques on my patients. Astonishingly, the great majority of them benefited, many of them straight away. But some of the things he taught were just ludicrous – they could not possibly be true. And this was reflected in his book – some things he wrote were just not scientifically valid at all. No wonder his views were not universally accepted. Clearly I needed to pursue this subject further.

Neither was I happy with some of the osteopathic teaching I looked at next. Obviously their results were a great deal better than mine had been before I developed my interest in the field. But some of what they said was just not compatible with proven scientific fact. And I found chiropractic teaching no more scientific. Both disciplines were lodged firmly in faith. I was intellectually lost. I did not know where to turn for guidance. Salvation came from an unexpected source.

To broaden my experience and understanding I had joined the appropriate medical association of those interested in the subject. I had attended numerous meetings, where I found a wide spectrum of excellence and nonsense – heavily loaded in favour of the nonsense side, or so I thought. After some time (with no specific training for it) I had been co-opted to teach for the association. This proved quite a revelation, as many of our teachers seemed to be short on the evidence side of the subject. In doing this, I met one man in particular who seemed to talk an awful lot of sense, and who was distinctly short on the waffle. This was refreshing indeed. And then at coffee time on one course a visiting Italian doctor asked me if I could organise a course at the University of Rome. His professor had explicitly asked him to explore this possibility. I was dumbfounded.

'Sit down, Dr Minelli. Don't move. I want you to discuss this proposition with my colleague, Dr Brown.'

I found Leonard chatting with a group of postgraduate students. I took him aside, told him what Dr Minelli had said, and asked him what he thought of the idea.

'We must go. There's no question about it. Lead me to him.'

After a brief discussion we agreed to discuss the whole project at the end of the day's work. Both Leonard and I found it hard to concentrate on what we were meant to be teaching. At the end of the day we agreed the basic format of the projected course. Dr Minelli seemed well pleased, and it was not long before we had our visit confirmed by his professor. Leonard and I spent much of the next six months devising a five-day course. Though we did not realise it at the time, this was the start of a seventeen-year cooperation between us, involving an enormous amount of fresh work and the publication of no fewer than eight books. But more of that later.

Now I found that I was spending more and more time dealing with back pain in the practice. The results were enormously encouraging. And then I had something of a setback. After I had successfully relieved Maggie's pain, she asked me to see her father. She brought him along, but I failed to help him at all – indeed if anything I made him rather worse. I was uncertain what to do – so I said so. Gordon agreed that he would see the great man in London – I could think of no other authority. I suggested that I might drive him there, so that I could be in on the learning side of it. So I did just that. I was horrified at what I saw – it seemed a quite barbaric assault on the poor chap and Gordon was made worse than ever. I did not enjoy my journey home. But one good thing came out of that unhappy event. I became even more critical of what I was doing myself.

Happily, events like Gordon's sorry tale were very rare. As I mentioned earlier my bank manager was a patient of mine, on account of a painful neck. When I had decided to build a brand new surgery I had needed his assistance over funding, so I had telephoned him.

'John,' he said, 'I'm so glad you rang. I've got a bit of a recurrence of my neck pain. If you could fit me in soon, perhaps we could talk about your proposal then.'

That seemed a great idea. He had come along that very evening. Sure enough, he had the same pain as he had suffered before. I thought it must have been something to do with his posture at work. I had got him onto the couch and moved his head about cautiously.

'Kenneth, I've heard about people having their arms twisted, but this is ridiculous. I am going to twist not your arm but your neck. It is all right about my loan, isn't it?'

'I think you had better do your stuff first, John. Then I will be in a better state to help. Or I hope I will be.'

Yes, Kenneth was pain-free, and I was soon free to go ahead with building my dream surgery.

Not long after the awful experience with Gordon, I failed to relieve a very nice girl of her low back pain. I made three attempts, but she was no better. I referred her to an orthopaedic surgeon. She had probably got a true disc protrusion. Months later I had a phone call from her, to thank me for my help.

'It is sweet of you to ring, but I'm afraid I failed to help you at all.'

'Oh I know, doctor, but you listened to me – and you tried.'

There was a lesson to be learned there.

One of the things I learned was that lumbar traction was sometimes very helpful. The main problem for many patients was that the ride to the hospital was often tedious, and the ride home frequently undid any good the traction might have done in the outpatient department. This was an indication for another little innovation on my part. I designed a portable traction apparatus, for use in the patient's home. Using this, rather than suffering the commonly damaging journey home, the patient could stay lying down after treatment – perhaps even overnight.

My invention was very simple, affording two hooks (held about eight feet apart when assembled) between which the chest harness and the pelvic harness were slung, together with a pulley and a butcher's scale. It could be laid down on the patient's own bed, without the need for any sort of fixing – other than to the patient. I got a friendly local garage owner to make the rigid part out of several sections of exhaust tubing. It packed away into a very manageable wooden box, easily stowed in the car, and it all fitted together very quickly. The harnesses were made by a local saddler. I was even invited to demonstrate it at a postgraduate meeting at my old teaching hospital.

The great day came, and I drove merrily up to London. I sat through the first lecture very happily. Then I was asked to speak out of turn, as the person who should have been speaking next had not yet arrived. Of course, I agreed. I rushed out to my car to collect the apparatus. Dashing up to the platform, I hastily got out my gear, assembling it with a certain amount of clanging. Before I could start to demonstrate the wretched thing, a voice from the back of the lecture theatre rang out loud and clear – it was a senior doctor from the Physical Medicine department.

'Christ. It's the bloody plumber.'

That was not my only delight over the traction apparatus. I spent some time driving in and out of town – after supper – to treat an elderly businessman. All went very well the first evening. On the second evening there was a great improvement. When I released Mr Tonkin from his second session of traction, he made an odd request.

'I assume you drink whisky. I wonder whether you would mind if I made a small experiment on you? Over there in the corner you will find a tray with three bottles on it. Each bottle is numbered, but not otherwise labelled. I would like to know what you think of each of them.'

'Mr Tonkin, I'm afraid I know very little about whisky – I just rather like it.'

'That is precisely why I ask you to tell me what you think of these three. Whisky blending is a most complex business, and it takes months before one can assess any change one has affected by altering the balance between different malts. I have devoted a lot of time to this matter. In fact it has been a hobby of mine for years. I want a totally unbiased view. Let us start with Number One. Would you be so kind as to do the honours? If you would help me prop myself up a bit perhaps we can sip them together.'

We spent some time sipping the three blends. Each time he wanted to know what I thought. They all seemed pretty good to me. But the last was quite different from any I had tasted before.

'Mr Tonkin, I think they are all delicious. I would not pick out either of the first two, but do tell me what the third one is. It is so light, so delicate, and it has an odd flavour which I just cannot place. It's really something special.'

'Doctor, you have just proved me right. I said I wanted an unbiased opinion. The third is a blend I have been working on for nearly eighteen months. The flavour you note comes from the iodine in the water of source. The Western Isles malts all have this distinctive flavour. Millions of years ago the islands were submerged under the sea. Today's peat bogs are based on seaweed – hence the iodine. I am marketing this next week. Oh, and thank you so much for your help – and please send me your bill straight away.'

I was rather late home, but it had been a most interesting evening. A week or so later I received his cheque – plus a whole case of the new whisky. Perhaps he was not just being generous – I never bought any other whisky until after his death, when the blend ceased to be marketed.

Whisky was not my sole tipple. As an integral part of biology, I had learned to make beer at school. Yes, the feeding, reproduction and waste disposal system of the yeast plant are certainly part of biology. And if you make it yourself you can adjust the strength and the bitterness to suit your own taste. So yes, I found time to do that as well – the ingredient cost being no more than two old pence a pint made it even more delicious. Of course I shared the odd pint with numerous patients.

For a short while I took on the additional task of postgraduate teaching in general practice. After attending an excellent course in London, I got involved in something new. It occurred to me that a tape-recording of what my trainee and his patient said to each other might be good material to discuss at the end of each session. This involved having to get the patient's agreement, but when I explained that the tape would be wiped clean after we had talked about it, no one ever declined. One of the things I had learned on my course had been that a patient is easily distracted by something moving – like the tape revolving. The answer must be to put the machine in the desk drawer, which remained slightly open leaving only an immobile microphone on the writing surface. I found this very helpful. But I did not pursue this for long. There were so many other things to do.

There was a brief period when I strayed right away from medicine. It all started when I discovered woodworm infestation in the house. The prospect of enormous bills for its treatment was worrying. I bought a book on timber decay and somehow found time to read it. I got more and more fascinated by what I read. Here was spelt out a specific form of therapeutics – applying a chosen chemical to kill the infecting organisms without doing harm to the host. This was applied medicine. I was doing it every day. Dozens of times. If they could do it, so could I. Not only did I treat my own property, but I went so far as to form a small company to offer sensible treatment of woodworm and dry rot to others – at a reasonable price. Maybe my new patients were already dead, but the principles were the same. Then I added chemical damp-courses, but that was not really medicine. It had to end – there just wasn't the time to keep it going.

After a while I was seeing some back patients at our house. One particular episode was quite unforgettable. After taking a careful history, for the second (and last) time in my life I repeated the same big mistake of years ago.

'Right, Mrs Daniels, just take off a few things.'

I finished writing her notes before looking up. There she stood, stark naked. Unlike the subject of my previous similar mistake, she was ravishingly beautiful, leaving me speechless for a moment. It was at this point that the door opened, and in walked my two-year-old daughter.

'Hello.'

Eva Daniels' reply was charming. She smiled very sweetly at the little girl.

'Hello.'

Hurrying the small intruder out of the room (this time locking the door behind her) I returned to my patient very embarrassed. I suggested a modest degree of dressing, and then dealt with her problem – very successfully. She was highly entertained by the whole unexpected drama. We both told of the event for years afterwards. It went down very well after a dinner party.

Time for more innovation. Like everyone else I knew, I had always advised patients with back problems to use a firm mattress. I did not think that putting a board under the existing one was very kind. And then I questioned the sense behind that advice. Doubting Thomas had to be my role model. If the patient were to lie on his back, then the firmer the mattress the more he would lie 'at attention'. The back of his head, his shoulder blades, his buttocks and his heels would be more or less in a straight line. But what happened when he turned onto his side? For example, his left side. His shoulders being the widest bit, his head would droop sideways – to the left. The next wide bit being his hips, his spine would sag between shoulders and hips – in the other direction – producing a bend to the right. Surely the firmer the mattress the worse strains would be put on the spine – unless he managed to sleep on his back all night. What was needed was a mattress which automatically changed in form with changes in posture – and gave uniform support the whole way.

So what about the water-bed? I saw several things wrong with that. Its cost was quite beyond the means of most of my patients, it was too heavy for some bedroom floors that I knew and (if it leaked) it might ruin the ceiling below. Also, if one rollicked about on it one might get sea-sick.

What about the inflated mattress, such as was often used in camping? The chief thing wrong with this seemed to be that if it was to keep hips and shoulders off the floor it had to be inflated pretty fully – to the extent that it was almost as bad as the board. I had an answer to this. This was to make a mattress cover deeper than most, with two or four partitions down the length of it (to provide a single or double mattress). Into each 'slot' one put an airtight tube, with several partitions across the width, each of which had four tiny holes in it. One inflated the tubes through a valve at one end – only sufficiently to make the mattress 'stand up' when not weight-bearing. This gave one a long narrow 'balloon' made up of six more or less cubic sections, with the ability for air to move from one section to the next – under pressure, *but slowly*.

Sit on the edge of the mattress, and the nearest tube would

slowly lower one's behind, progressively emptying one or two sections of that tube, at the same time as inflating those in its upper and lower sections. Lie in the middle of it and one's weight would be spread over two or three tubes. This would adjust the shape of the mattress, offering a uniform pressure at all levels – regardless of whether the patient lay on his back or his side. Perfect comfort with equal support along the length of the spine – within a few seconds of changing position.

I took out a patent – at some expense. I had a few made. They cost a bomb. I tried it out myself. It was blissfully comfortable. I tried it out on a few patients. They were without exception delighted with it. I failed to get a manufacturer to take it on. I gave up.

All the additional work I had taken on had to have an effect in the long run. I was doing two clinical jobs simultaneously, as well as thinking up all manner of new interests. Something had to give. As will be described in detail in Chapter 9, I discovered that my blood pressure was dangerously high. I had to decide whether I would run the very real risk of having a major stroke far too young, submit to life-long drug taking (of which I had an absolute horror), or change my way of life – and give up general practice. It was a difficult choice to make. Was I to abandon the majority of my patients or risk becoming one myself? I just had to change down a gear. I retired from general practice.

Though disappointing, there was still a lot more going on in my world. My trip to Rome had been a limited success, in spite of near disaster. Leonard and I had thought we would need a third member of the team if we were to manage the numbers Dr Minelli had suggested. Our choice was unfortunate. In six months Bertram had done no preparation for his role at all, saying he had been too busy and making a miserable showing on every count in Rome. He was also extremely rude to the Professor. Happily he had taken advantage of the course to make it the first step of a holiday, so Leonard and I flew home without him. Perhaps he was doubly fortunate – we might otherwise have done him grievous bodily harm.

On the plane we reviewed our days in Rome. First the two of us could manage very well on our own. Second the response from our hosts had been pretty encouraging, in that many doctors had shown great interest in what we had to offer. Third we were not going to waste the six months' slog of preparation – we would set up our own courses in England. We parted company at Heathrow with a pretty clear idea as to how we were going to proceed – totally independent of our national association. Within a fortnight I had drafted our first handbook and we had written the programme for our first course. Four months later I had written a second, complementary handbook. Out of near disaster we had started on a seventeen-year run of truly rewarding teaching.

It was early on in this process that I found myself chatting to an old friend, Professor Winston. He was perhaps my most un-favourite patient. This was because he was unbelievably bright, a professor of biochemistry who was also a veterinary surgeon and ran a very go-ahead research institute. He knew very much more of the scientific basis of medicine than I did. I had soon learned to ask him the normal value of this and that, before I commented on his own condition. Now I was showing him the two handbooks I had written.

'These are splendid, John, but they deserve better than their somewhat homespun appearance. I think you ought to publish a "proper" book. Look, I am going to be in the USA for a week or so. When I get back I shall be seeing my publisher. You must come and have lunch with us. I think he will be interested.'

More work. So it was that Leonard and I made sweeping changes to the handbooks, condensing them into one. I met the Professor's delightful publisher, Paul, who at once accepted the project. It was published in time for us to send a copy to each participant prior to our next course – with instructions to read it before they attended, preferably more than once. Little did we know it, but this was only the start of our publishing experience. Thank you, Professor Winston.

One of the doctors attending the course was a middle-aged GP from Hull. Alec was a very active participant, charmingly argumentative, and at the end of the course he was extremely appreciative of our efforts.

'I've been to a good many postgraduate courses over the years. Mostly they've been like going back to school. This one has been like going back to university. And the book is a wonderful addition to all the talk and the practical work. There's only one thing wrong with it.'

'You are more than kind, Alec. I am sure there are many things to criticise about it, but what have you got in mind?'

'It's that long word on the front. Too many folk will read that and put the book down. You need to write another book that will make them want to read this one.'

The long word was 'Manipulation'. But that was what the book was about. Leonard and I discussed the question at some length. In the end we agreed that Alec was right – there would be many doctors who would be put off by that word. What if we were to write a book on local examination of the back? I phoned Paul the next day, to enquire what he thought of Alec's comment.

'He's right. Write the other book – on local examination of the back. Everyone will read it – then they will want to read the first. You've got a publisher.'

We did as instructed. But this was not to be the end of the matter. In the meantime Leonard and I played our parts in the national association, and also in the international federation. This gave us wonderful opportunities for travel to many countries, in the course of which we saw a great many patients and met a wide variety of their doctors. It was a wonderful experience. Alec was not to know it, but he had started something – in the next few years we published three more books together and two more each independently. All this time I was working from home, at a small private hospital half an hour's drive away and in London.

It was time for more innovation. One day an old friend of mine telephoned to ask me whether I would like my own X-ray machine. He was the local radiologist.

'Ewart, you must be joking. I couldn't possibly afford that. And anyhow I wouldn't know what to do with it, if I had one.'

'Hang on a moment. No hasty decisions, please. Listen to this. One of my sector hospitals is about to replace a mobile set because it is rather old. In fact it has not been used very much and it is perfectly serviceable, but the NHS says it has to be replaced because of its date of birth – at a good many thousand pounds – at the taxpayer's expense. I think it will do all you need. If you want it, it's yours at metal scrap value – £200.'

This was too good to be true. Ewart was enormously helpful. He arranged that the two of us would collect it, on a trailer he borrowed, and that he would provide developing tanks and developer, which were currently taking up space in his garage. He helped me set it all up and he demonstrated how I should use it.

'But what if I get stuck, Ewart? I think I shall manage to take and develop some adequate pictures, but I may not have a clue what to make of them. You know what an ass I can be at times.'

'That's simple. You telephone me. If I can put you right over the phone, you have no problem. If I can't, then either you bring the difficult picture to me, or I come and look at it with you. It just depends upon how busy we each are.'

I did not go mad with this new toy, and I did not fall into the trap of thinking myself an expert radiologist. But it did permit me to improve the lot of a good many patients. Those who needed an X-ray got it – on the spot. No travelling miles into and out of hospital – no waits either for an appointment or to be dealt with when they got there. It took not much longer than the developer allowed. But it did something else for me – it gave me yet another idea.

At times differences of leg length are important to the patient. I had been taught to use a tape measure for this onerous task – measuring between the bony lumps at the inner side of the ankle and the front part of the hip. I found two things wrong with this – it was not a measure of leg length at all and in obese patients it was impossible to make anything like an accurate measurement as the bony points were hidden under mounds of fat. Osteopaths and chiropractors had introduced me to another way of estimating these differences – squatting behind the standing patient with the fingers lying along the hips and looking at a horizontal line of some sort. Again, while possibly useful, this was not a measure of differences in leg length at all. So what about X-ray? At least this would measure leg length accurately. If the pelvis were symmetrically formed this would be the answer to the problem. It is not. If one is looking for measurable indicators of what happens to the spine above the pelvis, one must look elsewhere.

It was Doubting Thomas who once more came to my rescue. Surely, any bends and strains on the (more or less erect) spine must be related to its not standing on a level base. If the base is aslant, the patient tends to lean over. The only way to correct this is for him to automatically bend his spine the other way – when it ought to be straight. And this means a compensatory bend in the other direction at a higher level – a scoliosis.

You could easily see a tilt of the upper surface of the sacrum on a front-view X-ray. The problem was how to measure the angle it made with the horizontal. A protractor was not well suited to small angles, and what use was it anyway? The answer seemed obvious. One drew just four lines on the X-ray – one vertical line through the highest point of each of the hip joints, one sloping line across the top of the sacrum, and a final horizontal line through where the sacral line crossed one of the two vertical ones. The use of simple trigonometry would show the effective difference in leg length – the tangent of the angle. One could measure the effective difference with ease – the distance on one of the vertical lines between the horizontal and sloping lines. It was so simple. I wanted to call it 'Paterson's index of sacral tilt' but I changed my mind. The 'lateral index of sacral tilt' would be more suitable – LIST. I just couldn't write a paper entitled 'PIST'.

Two patients were of particular interest in this context. Bernard was an Olympic speed skater. He came to me with a nasty lumbar problem. I was horrified to discover that he sported an effective leg length difference of 5.5 centimetres. This was gross.

'It's a good thing it's wrong the right way round, Bernard. If it were the other way you would fall over on your first bend. I bet you would. Try it in reverse.'

Another case was even more extraordinary. Wilfred was a village postman. He did his round on a bicycle. Again he had a low back problem. He too was very lop-sided. When I measured it, his effective leg length difference worked out at 6.5

centimetres. When his back pain had gone he asked me whether I thought he could resume his running. What running? Several years before he had joined his son in cross-country running – he was then in his early sixties. The son had tried to dissuade him, saying he was far too old, but his father insisted and from the very start left his son far behind. He was a natural. He really 'got the bug', ending up as number five in the world for the over-sixty-five marathon. He was astonished when I told him what I had found – he had no idea there was anything amiss.

My last resort with low back pain was to give the patient an epidural injection. Nature is good enough to provide a small hole just where the tail-bone joins the sacrum, which makes it quite easy to do – usually. I did many of these, but one recollection remains very vivid. My patient was a very pleasant neighbouring GP. He was near to retiring age and was substantially overweight, in spite of being a very heavy smoker. One very hot summer's afternoon he pleaded with me to come and give him an injection at home. I obliged. He was in a lot of pain, and we agreed that this was the best thing to do – indeed the only thing. We were in his sitting room, and with some difficulty he managed to lie on a very low couch. The little hole was very hard to find – his great collops of fat hid it. I was on my knees for an awful long time before I managed to do my job – sweating for two reasons. Moments later Walter sat up briskly.

'My God, John, I really thought I was going to die.'

'I am so sorry. I'm afraid it was a frightful job to get into the canal at all.'

'My dear fellow, it was not your performance that was troubling me. The pain in my back was so severe I dared not cough and I thought I would die of pneumonia. Now, thanks to you, I have no pain – I can cough to my heart's content. You won't have a fag, will you?'

7

Not All Plain Sailing

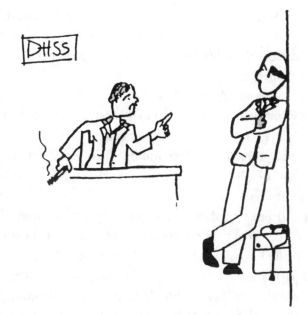

A life in medical practice is liable to take unexpected turns. Rare is he who does not run into some sort of trouble from time to time. And the troubles are just about as varied as the vast range of clinical problems he meets every day. It must be remembered that, however good he is and however hard he tries, no doctor can satisfy all his patients all the time. And it is not only patients who may initiate problems. Not very long after Maurice and I had been joined by a third partner, Dick, we were to enjoy a visit by the Regional

Medical Officer more than we anticipated. Such visits were not usually very rewarding – indeed, to the busy doctor they seemed an awful waste of time. Of course it is reasonable to have some sort of eye kept on what is going on in the world of general practice, particularly if the system is lodged in the State. But those deputed as watchdogs should be both well-informed and well-intentioned.

This time it was different. The Regional Medical Officer was due to meet us at two. Mary was busy in the hall when the bell rang some minutes before this time. For some reason she was sure it was Maurice. Snatching the door open, she popped her head round the jamb.

'You're too early, Maurice.'

Terribly embarrassed, she ushered the startled Dr Black into my study and called me from the kitchen. Happily, both Maurice and Dick joined us very soon. These routine visits usually started with examination of the dangerous drugs register – a perfectly legitimate routine chore. That done, this time the Regional Medical Officer seemed to have other things on his mind – it was almost as if he had a mission. He appeared to delight in hauling us over the coals for a practice we all three openly shared. To stave off serious chest infections in the winter, we routinely gave chronic bronchitic patients a prophylactic course of antibiotics in the autumn. We three agreed that it had been shown to be a pretty effective policy. In Dr Black's view it was an unjustifiable waste of public money. It must be stopped. We argued that, apart from commonly doing individuals good, it was an effective way of reducing hospital admissions in this group of patients. Rather than wasting money, it thus saved the taxpayer a very substantial sum. Dr Black was not impressed. We seemed to be getting nowhere. It was young Dick who got us out of trouble.

'Dr Black, I wonder whether you have read this recent paper on the subject from the Brompton Hospital – surely the Mecca of chest diseases?'

He waved an open journal in the general direction of our visitor.

'I'm afraid not. I really have not had the time to read much recently.'

'What a pity – I think you really ought to read it. It reports on a very large study over a two-year period, and its statistical validity is impeccable. It presents decisive evidence on the value of what we are doing – and in particular stresses the savings derived from the practice, quite apart from any direct benefit to the patient. Forgive me for asking, but have you any experience of general practice, Dr Black?'

'Oh, yes – more than twenty years of it.'

'May I ask why you left this fascinating field?'

'A most interesting question. I am afraid I have another appointment elsewhere. I really must be off. Good afternoon to you all.'

With that he had left – driving off into the sunshine on that chilly winter day. Well done, Dick. Of course, we continued to help our patients and to save taxpayers' money. Our local hospitals were delighted at their minimised work-load, too.

Tragically, one of my professional neighbours died at an early age from liver failure. His was a sad case indeed. A chronic alcoholic, 'L' had been a patient of mine for some years before his death. To be frank, his professional standards were very low. The whole of the top storey of his lovely old house was devoted to the rearing of turkeys, while he lived in some squalor below – with his wife and two scruffy dogs. I think his wife was a nurse. When he was too drunk to see patients, she would see them on his behalf, telling them he was out visiting patients, quite illegally signing sickness certificates and prescriptions in his name. From time to time she would tell patients wanting to be visited that I was on call – although no such arrangement had ever been made. In spite of this, most of his patients loved him dearly. He was indeed a very warm, caring man.

Not long before his death I heard the story behind his addiction. Winning two major undergraduate prizes, he had been a very promising young doctor. He had served in good junior posts in his teaching hospital before joining the Army as a medical officer towards the end of the war. He had been madly in love with a girl, and they had made plans to settle down together at the end of his military service. Her dramatic, avoidable death started him on his drinking habit, which rapidly became a serious addiction. He was running away from an agonising piece of history. In the end it killed him. I was glad that he had managed to tell someone his story. At heart he was such a decent man. Should I have reported his gross inadequacy to the authorities? Should I have 'sneaked' on his wife's dangerous activities? Should Dr Black have spent more time with him than with us?

I saw another case of liver failure. Eric and his wife ran a small store in 'my' main village. They worked very hard and made quite a decent living out of it. By the time he was fifty Eric was doing very well. This time I never found out what triggered it, but he descended into alcoholism, like 'L'. He rapidly became quite ill. Nothing helped him and he deteriorated steadily. Eventually I sent him to a very progressive surgeon, who decided that a liver transplant should be attempted. But even that did not stem Eric's decline and he died during the operation. At least everything possible had been tried – one cannot win all the tricks. His widow was heartbroken and left the area shortly afterwards.

There was an odd sequel to this tale. Months later I read a report in one of the journals of what was claimed to be the first liver transplant to be performed in the country – it was a wonderful success. Yes, it was the same surgeon who had done his best for Eric. But why did he choose to deceive his readers? As he very well knew, it was not the first liver transplant, it was the second – the first had failed, the patient dying in the operating theatre.

A funny as much as sad story concerned a farmer who was allergic to bee venom. David insisted, against all advice, on keeping bees. Ten or a dozen hives. What was all the fuss about? Bee stings were something he lived with. He was sure he would be all right. An excellent farmer when in going order, now and again things went a bit wrong – when he found himself the quarry of a swarm of angry bees. Usually it all went away quite soon. Not every time. One day his wife called me in great anxiety, saying that David had been badly stung and had had one of his attacks in the cowshed, and that she was going straight back to him. She had left the front door open. I could come in and find my own way through the kitchen.

Happily I knew the house well. It was a lovely old red-brick farmhouse with Dutch gables and I always thought it would have suited me very well. It was dark and very cold that evening as I made my way through the house, across the yard and into one of the two large cattle sheds. High up and towards the far end, there hung a low-wattage lightbulb, shedding no more than a glimmer of light in the enormous space. There were cows in almost every stall, munching away very happily in the gloom. They did not seem to care either about the dimness or about my arrival.

In the last stall on the left was a picture reminiscent of a Christmas crib. There sat Betty on a heap of straw, looking remarkably serene, with the unconscious David's head in her lap. The inadequate bulb made a somewhat anaemic Star of Bethlehem. I felt as if I were meant to be a wise man. I was certainly neither a shepherd nor a king. Back to the job in hand. This was no place to deal with the patient. But how on earth was I to get him into a more suitable environment? Putting my bag down on the distinctly mucky floor of the shed, I gave him a quick injection and dashed back into the yard. On my way in I had noticed a wheelbarrow near to the cowshed. Now I emptied it of its load of cow dung before bringing it inside. Somehow Betty and I managed to get the unconscious David into the barrow and I proceeded along the ill-lit aisle of munching cows and across the yard with my unaccustomed and distinctly smelly load. Betty carried my mucky bag. As we were about to heave him out he regained consciousness.

'Bugger they bees! Bugger they bees!'

Betty and I collapsed with laughter. I saw him to bed before going home to share the tale with Mary. Needless to say, David went on keeping bees. They produced some lovely honey – and yes, on one occasion I made some delicious mead from some of it.

I have already described some of my dealings with the rhinoceros-nosed Mrs Burdett. One year I was to be off duty from finishing work on Christmas Eve for the rest of the Christmas holiday. Although it meant deviating from my normal route, I deliberately left Mrs Burdett to the end of my visiting list. She was her usual generous self, and I set off for home almost at dusk, my car full of Brussels sprouts and the rest, leaving Alfred with a handsome supply of his 'lumbagoa tablets'. About halfway home I was passing through a small copse, where the road had had no sun all day, when on a bend I hit a patch of black ice. I lost control completely. I came to a halt with my front wheels in the copse hedge, my rear wheels on the grass verge, and my door above a deep ditch – its bottom covered over with ice. There were sprouts everywhere. As luck would have it, there was a public phone box not three hundred yards away and, once I had managed my rather precarious escape from the car, I summoned help. The local breakdown man turned up remarkably quickly. He thought it was hilariously funny.

'That's a bloody silly place to park a car, doctor. I'd 'ave thought you'd 'ave known better. Look, it's a bit chilly 'ere. I think I'd better run you 'ome first and see to the car after that.'

Bless him, he did just that. I got home for my brief Christmas holiday a trifle later than anticipated – without the sprouts – and my slightly modified car was back in action in time for me to go back to work as intended.

There must have been something about Mrs Burdett's village. It was here that I had a bit of a contretemps with Sid. He was for ever trying to get me to give him sickness certificates to enable him to go off on expeditions – regardless of whether he was unfit for work or not. We fell out over this on more than one occasion. He was a real scrounger. Stopping at a house further up the village one day, I was warned to be very careful – Sid had been down to the Black Bear, had had a bit too much to drink and had been seen striding round the village with a loaded shotgun, 'looking for that bloody doctor'. Happily, he did not find me.

Remembering the occasion when I had had such difficulty doing an epidural injection for my rather obese colleague, I proposed the same treatment for a new patient, Mrs Asher. She was distinctly apprehensive about it, so I explained everything to her carefully, and we agreed that we should try it. There seemed little else I could offer. Her husband sat without saying a word, just watching the proceedings. Having described the procedure to her, I got her installed on the couch – no kneeling this time. I washed my hands and prepared the injection. Just as I turned towards her, Mrs Asher twisted round in great haste, a look of horror on her face.

'Doctor, I must see the needle.'

With that she lost her balance and crashed onto the floor. Her silent husband and I picked her up, happily finding no real damage. I did not proceed with my chosen therapy. For some reason she never came back to see me.

I have reason to remember that couch well – in a number of contexts. I bought it because of its adjustability – not because its cover was bright orange. It served me well. Lizzy Wood was in her late fifties, distinctly overweight and very talkative. She was a pleasant sort of person. She had come to me with pain in the right side of her chest. I had taken a careful history, in view of her age asking about other conditions, and particularly whether she had ever broken any bones (possibly as a result of osteoporosis). I had gone on to examine her, when I had found clear physical signs suggesting that simple vertebral manipulation was the treatment of choice. Explaining this to Mrs Wood, I installed her on my lovely orange couch. I used a manoeuvre I had used many times before. She screamed with pain.

'You've broken my rib, doctor!'

'Nonsense, Mrs Wood, I couldn't possibly have done so.'

'Oh yes you have. I've got a congenital cyst there – it's been broken twice before.'

Though I certainly failed to help sometimes, that was only the second occasion I remember when I actually made anybody worse. When I asked Mrs Wood why she had told me on direct questioning that she had had no fractures in the past, her answer was surprising.

'I didn't think a rib mattered, doctor.'

'I'm so sorry, Mrs Wood, but if you had told me when I asked you, I would never have used the technique I did, and you would not be in trouble like this. Let's see what we can do about the fracture – at least I can improve that with a simple injection and some painkillers. It will be a while before it is healed, I'm afraid – the best part of three weeks – perhaps more.'

Happily, we parted the best of friends. The lesson to be learned here was that it was not enough to take a scrupulous history – one had to gain honest answers to straight questions. I hope Mrs Wood got the same message.

I only once had a similar calamity. I gave a simple injection to a patient who was allergic to the local anaesthetic I gave him. I had asked Ted Birch whether he had any allergies. He had said no. Moments after giving him the injection, he suffered anaphylactic shock. After reviving him I asked him if he had ever had anything like it before.

'Oh, yes. I forgot to mention it. I've had trouble with dentists for years – they always have to give me gas.'

'Mr Birch, I asked you about that. You said no. All's well now, but please don't forget in the future.'

How could anybody be so silly as not to tell the truth, when asked a straight question? What a chump. And what a good thing I made a habit of always being prepared for the worst, so the antidote was at hand.

Ellie Bentley was an attractive, intelligent, middle-aged woman who lived in a rather lovely, solitary, thatched cottage with her large and very domineering husband. She was never ill. One day her husband demanded that I visit her. He seemed put out that I wanted to know something about the case on the phone. There seemed no point in arguing, so in due course I went along. I was not received with good grace, and Mr Bentley insisted on pacing up and down the landing while I saw Ellie in the bedroom. With the door wide open, this was a trifle disturbing. Ellie was quite ill. I wished I had been able to get more information about her on the phone – I would have certainly re-routed my afternoon visits so as to see her earlier. I decided that she must be admitted to hospital for further investigation without delay. On the landing Mr Bentley was not best pleased with my suggestion.

'You should have been here long ago. It's about time you GPs did your jobs properly. My wife's not going into any bloody hospital.'

'Mr Bentley, your wife is ill – she needs to go into hospital for investigations which cannot be done here. What is more, she needs to go in now.'

'You do your bloody job, or I'll throw you downstairs, you little git.'

We clearly had three problems here. A seriously sick patient who needed urgent admission to hospital, a near lunatic who needed calming down, and a doctor at risk of grievous bodily harm. This was no time for discussion. With the very aggressive husband towering over me, I took a gamble.

'All right, Mr Bentley – carry on then.'

His mouth dropped open as he sat down heavily on a chair. I heaved an audible sigh of relief.

'May I use your telephone, please? I need to get on with my job.'

All went smoothly after that encounter. The patient was

admitted and sorted out, while I was able to get on with my round – if a trifle shaken. Happily I never saw Mr Bentley again.

A near neighbour of the turkey-raising, alcoholic 'L' was his local parson. He was not a patient of mine. Perhaps I was spared something. But 'L' had described his eccentric patient's odd behaviour to me one day. The good rector was in sharp disagreement with his bishop. He lived in a beautiful old house, topped with the lovely local frost-split stone tiles. It was true that it had not been well maintained. The parson had found a slight leak in his roof, and demanded that it be attended to immediately. The bishop was not willing to do anything about the roof – yet. The argument escalated rapidly. It was resolved by the parson. He took a ladder to his chilly loft, bearing a yard broom. He then proceeded to jab the broomstick between the rafters again and again, smashing a considerable number of tiles and leaving a gaping hole. He then rang the bishop to complain that the leak was worse. I had met the parson once, and I was not entirely surprised to hear the tale. He had seemed dafter than most.

I seem to have an odd effect on parsons. Some I found delightful, as patients as well as people, but I have to admit that I found it difficult to be charitable about them all. One was a foxy little man, who expected his parishioners to be at his beck and call in many situations and on many occasions. He ordered the Women's Institute about, regardless of what they wanted to do for their own organisation. He demanded that the Parish Council supply him with a car, rather than just contributing to its running costs. He upset the longstanding pillars of the local church, almost without exception. He was assiduous in visiting the sick, though what degree of comfort he might have brought was uncertain. It was over this matter that we came to real disagreement. He marched into my surgery one day and wasted no time in pleasantries.

'I'm not sick, doctor. I just want you to do something for me. I would like you to give me a copy of your visiting list each day, so that I can the better minister to the sick. And I would like an idea of what I am to find in each one of them – an outline of their problems.'

'I am frankly a bit surprised at your request. My patients decide when they want me to visit them. They alone make that choice – and put in the request to me. I owe them a guarantee of privacy. On that basis I could not possibly give you information as to their state of health, let alone a copy of my visiting list. I'm sorry – it's just not on.'

'I really had hoped for better collaboration from you, doctor. All I'm asking for is your visiting list. What's wrong with that?'

'If my patients wish me to see them, they ask me. I see no reason why they may not do the same if they want you to visit them. I am sorry, but it would be quite unethical for me to do as you ask.'

Not a happy encounter. Too bad if the parson did not love me very much. I was not prepared to inflict his perhaps unwelcome presence upon my patients.

A very far cry from this chap, the parson in another village was quite extraordinary. Stephen had taken holy orders rather late in life, having farmed in Kenya for a good many years. I have seldom met a more genuine and approachable man. He had a wonderful manner with his parishioners, talking to them totally naturally in terms they understood. He was full of humour, as well as being a man of real compassion. I was always glad of an excuse to stop and talk with him. His flock respected him and found his easy, homely way most comforting. He was an exceptional country parson, and he so obviously loved what he was doing. But I shall come back to Stephen shortly.

When the demanding old parson left the parish, I heaved something of a sigh of relief. I never heard any patient say anything nice about his stay there – which was mercifully brief. But then I never asked. His replacement was temporarily installed in a small house right opposite my new surgery, waiting until renovations had been completed to the rather splendid old rectory. In fact it was the house I had had digs in with the worthy Gwen, when I had first come to the practice. One afternoon I shall not forget for a long time. I had called into the surgery to do some urgent dispensing, before carrying on with my busy round. It was at about three o'clock that the phone rang. It was the new parson from across the road. He must have seen my car.

'Is that the doctor? Good. This is the Reverend Terence Bertrand. I would like you to call at the temporary rectory, please. You know, just across the road.'

'Yes, Mr Bertrand, this is the doctor. May I ask what is your problem? I am afraid I am a bit tied up at the moment. It's not urgent, is it?'

'Oh, there's no problem, doctor. I just wanted you to look in to take over the family's care. I have our medical cards ready.'

'Could you please bring your cards over to the surgery? It will be open again at six. I am just about to go out again, to finish my rounds.'

'Oh no, doctor. We never go to the surgery.'

I got the distinct impression that I should not get involved with this family. Perhaps he felt I was less than welcoming. No cards arrived from across the road. Happily he went elsewhere, and I was spared this. But a few days later I met him coming out of the village grocery store. His large, portly figure blocked the doorway. I bade him good day. He looked me up and down and, without a word, turned and walked away. I felt sure that I was wise in distancing myself from this sort of behaviour.

A while later I had a laugh with my dear parson friend Stephen about this episode. He found it difficult to believe my story.

'I've only met the chap once. I can't say I warmed to him greatly, but this is outrageous. Do you want me to go and kick his arse?'

'Thanks a lot, Stephen, but I don't think that will be necessary. He has already gone elsewhere for his family's care. But I knew you would appreciate the tale.'

Between the three of us in the practice, we covered a long stretch of the Great North Road. Traffic accidents were not uncommon. Sometimes these were serious, sometimes relatively trivial, but always they disrupted the routine work. On the whole they were rather a bore. One day, towards the end of my morning surgery, I had a call to a bad accident. A big vehicle had slid into a ditch. It was deep winter, and the road conditions were pretty bad. With a quick apology to my current patient, I grabbed my emergency bag and drove to the scene of the accident as fast as the road would allow. It was seriously slippery and there was a biting wind.

Arriving at the scene, I found a large furniture van in the ditch, leaning perilously against a low branch of an elm tree. Underneath there was said to be a cyclist. The van driver was unhurt, but deeply in shock. The police were at the scene, but neither the ambulance nor the heavy breakdown team had yet arrived. There was no time to be lost. Leaving my bag on the verge, I managed to crawl under the skirt of the van, where I found the cyclist in a lot of pain – with a broken thigh.

'Hang on a moment. There's not much I can do for the leg just now, but I'll give you an injection for the pain. I'll be back in a jiffy.'

Crawling back onto the verge, I filled a syringe and crawled back again, trying not to dirty the needle on my way. I think I managed that, and anyway the patient was very grateful.

'Thank you so much, doctor. I really thought I'd had it.'

'Not this time. The injection should make things a little better. The ambulance should be here any moment. I'm afraid your bike seems to be in a worse state than you are.'

As I began to emerge for the second time, the branch of the tree snapped and the van settled a fraction lower. I thought I was going to be trapped with my patient till we were both rescued. Somehow I managed to wriggle out. Then the ambulance arrived. I was very glad to see it. But there was no way they could get the poor cyclist out until the heavy breakdown team had lifted the van a little. They arrived within a minute of the ambulance, and I left them to it. As I got back into my car I realised that I was wearing a brand new suit – first time on. It was ruined – filthy and with a great rent in it.

Perhaps the greatest drama in my professional life was in the case of Mrs Bull. She was a rather grand lady. She and her husband, Wilfred, had lived in the East for many years, where they had enjoyed numerous privileges. She expected this happy state to be continued in retirement in England. Unfortunately she became very ill. I referred her to an excellent surgeon in the nearby hospital. After undergoing surgery for her complaint, she needed daily dressings so my delightful district nurse went in each day. I needed to check on her slow progress rather less frequently. Although she was happy to drive three times as far to her hairdresser, Mrs Bull adamantly declined to come to see me. Like a chump, I accepted her demand.

One day the district nurse was attending to her rather slow-healing wound, when Mrs Bull stopped her.

'Nurse, I don't want the doctor to know about this.'

With that, she telephoned from her bedroom to make an appointment with another consultant – very much further away. Sensible and loyal lass that she was, the nurse came to see me. She was unhappy about it, but she felt that she ought to put me in the picture. Quite right, too. Clearly Mrs Bull did not trust me. But why had she not waited a few minutes until the nurse had gone, rather than involving her in demanding secrecy? Very odd. The only solution was for me to have her removed from my list of patients. I formally requested this the same day. It was the second of but two such requests I made over twenty-five years.

A week or so later I was busily engaged in my morning surgery when Wilfred Bull burst into my consulting room, through the door marked 'private'. I was in the middle of seeing a very surprised patient.

'It isn't true. You can't mean it. What the hell do you mean by taking my wife off your list? You'll put her back immediately.'

I very firmly escorted the fuming Mr Bull out of my room through the door he had left open, telling him that he must wait until I had finished with my current patient. He could use the waiting room, if he liked. He went on shouting, but I left him to it and shut the door. I returned to apologise to my startled patient for this wretched interruption. When she had left I sat for a moment wondering why he had been so furious. It seemed to me quite out of proportion. Going into the waiting room, I asked the other waiting patients whether I might deal with Mr Bull out of turn. Obviously sensing that I was in a difficult situation, they readily accepted this suggestion. Then I tried to find out why he was so furious. He ranted on for quite a while and was very angry when I declined to change my decision. At last I got rid of him and returned to my job. It was a most unpleasant encounter.

It was only later that I discovered the real reason for his outburst. What I did not know was that he was not only a member of the appropriate council, he was its chairman, and my request for removal of his wife from my list had been heard by the meeting he was chairing. Poor man, I felt quite sorry for him – it must have been an awful shock. And he was really a very decent chap at heart. Days later I received a most obnoxious letter from one of their sons. I ignored it.

One scare I could have done without was in London, where I was then working two days a week. This was after I had left general practice to concentrate on back pain. The very handsome big house was rather grand, and my room was right at the back. Everyone else had finished work, and I was tidying up before the long drive home. I heard a ring at the front door. Surely nobody could have an appointment at this hour? I went to the door and opened it.

'Are yer a bloody doctor? I need some cocaine.'

'I'm afraid that sort of thing is not in my line. I deal with nothing but back pain.'

'You're a doctor, ain't yer? I need a prescription. Understand?'

This man was distinctly aggressive and pushed his way into the hallway. There was nobody in the waiting room – there was not a sound to be heard upstairs. I imagined that the whole house was empty. I thought it was probably best to take him to my consulting room, to see if I could settle things down a bit. Try as I might, he got more and more aggressive, and I was fully expecting to have to use my wartime unarmed combat skills in self-defence. I was getting very worried. There was a tentative knock on my door.

Without waiting for a reply a slender little woman came in. She was a colleague's secretary who had been working late in the next room. She had heard the mounting row and came to get me out of trouble. She turned to the intruder.

'I think I can help. Come along with me.'

With that she took my visitor by the arm and led the lout away, leaving me utterly astounded. Within a very few minutes she was back, serenity itself.

'How on earth did you cope with that one, Eleanor? And thank you very much indeed for preserving me from a fate worse than death.'

'Oh, I just happen to be rather involved with drug addiction – in spite of working part-time for an orthopaedic surgeon. And it was really quite simple to get him unwound. It's a very different scene, isn't it?'

I was full of admiration for this girl. I was also full of shame that I had not handled the matter better myself.

At about the time of this incident I was also working one day a week at a small private hospital not far from home. I had been asked by a consultant gynaecologist to see a patient with persistent pain in her tail. When I arrived she was being X-rayed, so I had to wait a few minutes. In the waiting room there was a very pleasant man, who turned out to be a consultant psychiatrist from some way away. He was waiting for his wife to have a blood test done. We discovered that we had several things in common, including having served in Burma during the war. Our chat was interrupted by my old friend, Ewart, who came to tell me that my patient had had her X-ray and was back in her room. I thanked Ewart and turned to my new-found friend.

'Well, it was very pleasant talking to you. I must go now. I have work to do.'

Gone was his ready smile – the psychiatrist looked very solemn, as he shook me by the hand.

'I hope you realise that work is a four-letter word.'

I was not really looking forward to seeing this patient. When I had earlier asked the gynaecologist what her problem was, he had at first seemed almost lost for words. His ultimate reply I shall never forget.

'Oh, she's a pain in the arse with a pain in her arse.'

I soon found that his appraisal had been pretty sound. Everything was wrong. For a start, the gynaecologist was an uncaring, clumsy fool, the nurses were incompetent and rude, the bed was hideously uncomfortable and the food was disgusting. I was not looking forward to dealing with this lady. Added to that, it turned out that I was to have the dubious privilege of manipulating her tail-bone. She did not enjoy this very much – neither did I. I made my escape as soon as I could, fully expecting to be added to her list of moans.

The following Wednesday I arrived at the hospital to find the worthy gynaecologist waiting for me at the door.

'John, what the hell did you do to Moaning Minnie?'

'Oh dear, Norman, did I do her a mischief?'

'You certainly did not. She is a wholly different person. I am first-class, the nurses are kind, caring and efficient, the bed is heavenly and the grub is delicious. And as for you, the sun shines out of you know where.'

The patient was indeed very much better. But this was not to prove the end of my day. For the second time in my life, I skidded on black ice on my way home. This time I was driving a little sports car, which was said to be mid-engined. In fact the engine weight was only inches in front of the rear axle. This left too little weight on the front wheels for good steering. On icy roads it was not easily controllable. Unlike my Christmas Eve adventure, this time there was no ditch, so I sailed through a fairly young hedge into a grassy field. When I came to a halt, I found that the driver's door was badly damaged and I could not open it. Scrambling out the other side, I saw the extent of the damage – the car was seriously modified. But the engine was still running. If I came in that way, I could go out that way. Thank goodness the field was not ploughed. I swung round in a wide loop, aiming very carefully, and returned to the main road through the hole I had just made.

It was when I got home that the day really reached its climax. To be on the safe side, I stopped at the top of the drive, locked the car and started down the snowy slope. Yes, I slipped over, tobogganing down the drive on my back, preceded by my tobogganing bag. Mary wondered what could possibly go wrong next.

8

No Settled Abode

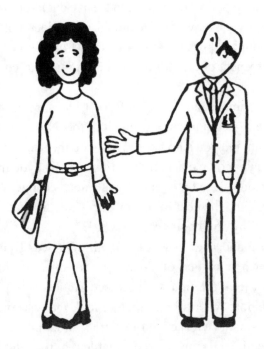

In the course of our life together, Mary and I certainly seemed to move house an awful lot. In the mad rush of getting out of the army, into medical school, into marriage and starting a family, the chance of settling down did not seem high. We more or less camped in three different flats in London before an odd thing happened. At a Commando reunion in the Porchester Hall I met an old friend, a fellow subaltern in No. 1 Commando, Frank Tucket.

We reminisced happily over a beer or two, catching up on each other's news since parting company in Burma, four years before. During our discussion on many topics, Frank really surprised me.

'John, why on earth do you stooge around paying rents to total strangers who don't give a toss about you, when you could just as well own your own place?'

'Don't be a chump, Frank. I managed to save damn-all from my army pay and my ex-service educational grant does not run to mortgages. I couldn't possibly buy a place – I have no capital at all and little prospect of any for an awful long time to come – if ever.'

'You're the chump, John. Since I left No.1 I have been working as an estate agent – and jolly interesting it is, too. Not a bad living, either. I bet I can find you a house and find you the necessary loan for you to have your own place. It doesn't matter that you may not stick around in one place for ever – if you want a change, you sell one property to fund the next. It must work. After all, that's how I make a living. Why don't you give it a whirl?'

I was dumbfounded at how easy it all sounded. But it did seem very much a matter of dreaming. In spite of that, the next weekend I took the time to go to see Frank's set-up in the suburbs of London. After a brief chat he took me just round the corner to see a small Victorian end-of-terrace brick house. Just to give me an idea. It had a tiny shelf of a garden in front and quite a long, narrow strip behind. Enough for quite a lot of vegetables. The little hallway was narrow, with a reasonably sized living room on the right which had a quite attractive bay window. A staircase went up opposite the front door, there was a tiny dining room behind the living room, with a window to the back garden, and a kitchen down the passage running between the stairs and the dining room. Upstairs there were two bedrooms and a bathroom.

It was rather dark and miserable looking, but that could be changed with a little paint and some cheerful curtains.

I thought our little family could manage there for a while anyway. I arranged for Mary to come and have a look. She agreed that it would at least start us off, so I took Frank's advice and took the plunge. Frank arranged the necessary loan. I bought our first house – for eight hundred and fifty pounds, freehold.

We settled in very happily, the only real problem being that I was so seldom there. Before I qualified, at weekends or in the evenings, I often used to walk along to a small cottage hospital, just up the hill. There I would watch the houseman doing routine things around the place – sometimes playing a more active role, helping in some way or another. Occasionally I used to give simple anaesthetics. Not legitimate, as the boss was not an official anaesthetics supervisor, but he was pretty watchful and I was very careful. The result of this was that, when it came to taking my final examinations, I had exceeded the required number of supervised anaesthetics by five times. Instead of twenty I had given one hundred. But I kept quiet about that.

Once I had qualified, I was at home even less. And, of course, the peace was shattered on the occasion my specs were smashed. Then, during my few months in Paddington I actually lived at home – and worked almost reasonable hours. When I decided to settle in country practice it was time to move on.

We sold our little home, making what I thought was an enormous profit – we got eleven hundred pounds for it. And then we had a small break while we lived in the old rectory, with the smelly Petter-engined water pump I mentioned earlier. Just for a little while we did not have a mortgage, but that happy state was not to last long. We had only gone to the rectory so as to be together while we looked for something permanent.

There was one property we did not buy. I fell in love with it at first sight. It was only a matter of a couple of hundred yards away from the cottage where I was later to be threatened with being thrown downstairs by the aggressive Mr Bentley. It was a large Georgian rectory, very elegant in style. It was most spacious and had four bedrooms, plus two attics. To one side there was an enormous garage that would have held a fleet of cars, while to the other side there was a substantial three-bedroomed semi-detached residence of the same vintage. The garden was charming, added to which there was a large, walled kitchen garden. All sorts of lovely fruits would be cascading down these walls in a few months' time. Around this were ten acres of grazing land – rented to a local farmer. And further towards the village the property included a pair of rather charming little thatched cottages, also rented out. The whole lot was for sale – at fifteen hundred pounds.

I wanted that property very much indeed, even though it probably needed quite a lot spending on it. I could not have it for one reason alone. The regulations of the NHS were such that the partners in the practice needed to live within a mile of each other – otherwise mileage payments would be calculated from each of our abodes, rather than from the practice centre. Our largest population was four miles from the present practice centre. A move to this lovely old rectory would have caused a substantial loss of mileage allowance – nothing would have been payable for the large number of patients currently qualifying for two or three mileage units each. This represented a considerable part of the practice income. Bill and I just could not afford such a loss of revenue. I really do not love bureaucracy.

Another thing endeared this house to me. It was a story of Robert's, from his very early days. As something of a new boy, he had been called by the rector to see a serving maid. On arrival he had been ushered up to the girl's room by the housekeeper. Dealing with the case in his usual methodical and down-to-earth manner, Robert had come downstairs, only to be met by the housekeeper hovering in the hall.

'Doctor, before you go the rector would like to have a word with you.'

This was not the happiest of prospects for Robert. He had come here to see a patient, not on a social mission. And it was not 'his' church either. He would very much rather get on with his visiting round. He had been ushered into the splendid study. It was pure Pickwick. This man was the last of a long line of rectors – the church was about to economise by not replacing him, which accounted for the availability of the property. The good rector was sitting comfortably at his desk.

'Oh, doctor, do sit down. I am sure you are busy. I won't keep you a moment. I have one small question only. What wine would be best for the patient?'

It was our landlord who suggested we might look at it. In a nearby village, less than a mile from Robert and Nora, the publican was giving up and his landlady was offering the little pub for sale. Apart from a few locals coming in for an evening beer, there was virtually no trade. It was a rather pretty thatched cottage on the corner of the tiny village green, with a pair of ugly brick barns beyond it. But it was not in very good shape and we soon discovered that it had no main drains and only a solitary main water tap in an outhouse – and no mains electricity either. On the face of it not very suitable for the doctor's family. It would certainly need a lot spending on it. When we went to have a look, we discovered that the garden was almost half an acre and there was also a small paddock going with it, perhaps a hundred and fifty yards down the lane – another one and a half acres. Already we were dreaming of children's ponies.

It was very tempting. We went mad and made an offer. Much to our surprise, Mrs Cowley accepted. Maybe it had something to do with the fact that she and her husband were patients of Robert's. Maybe we had offered too much. What mattered was that the price was agreed. And then the local solicitor told me something very odd. That funny little pub had a full licence – if the Justices were to approve its transfer to other premises, the licence would be a saleable article. He felt sure that the local brewery would be interested. Would I like him to apply on my behalf for a temporary transfer of the license? Yes, of course. On paper I was soon a licensed victualler – if only for a few weeks. Unlike the Archbishop of York (who was some years later to hold a licence, so that he might sell wines from the crypt of York Cathedral) I never sold a drop of anything. I bought the property for fifteen hundred pounds, and soon after sold the licence to the brewery for one hundred and twenty pounds.

The sale of the licence paid a delightful local builder to build a septic tank in engineering brick, bring the water into the house and give us a proper kitchen and a real bathroom. Dobby Fordson was such a nice man. He ran his own small building business in the next village, with the enormous help of his marvellous wife, Elspeth. There was nothing in the building trade that Elspeth could not do – digging, concreting, bricklaying, roofing, plumbing, wiring, she had even at times worked as a steeplejack. And she kept Dobby under pretty good control, too. Between them they made our new home very habitable – with great good humour and at very reasonable cost. Maybe Dobby's pipes did run a little out of true, but they took water where it was needed – without any leaks. Later he was to make the two barns into habitable dwellings.

But before that we had the cottage re-thatched. Percy Pettigrew was another patient, this time from 'my' half of the practice. He certainly worked hard, and with meticulous attention to symmetry. He replaced the whole thatch with lovely fen reeds, finishing it off with a big kiss just below where the chimney came through the ridge – for our elder son. What a delightful gesture. With fen reed, Percy told me, the thatch would last at least one hundred years – it would see us both out.

Our next two daughters were born in that cottage. The first one properly organised and conducted, the second in so much of a rush that I actually delivered her myself, before the midwife arrived. That was not quite what we had intended. At least I was no longer a beginner and miraculously I was there at the right time – it was at the weekend, and I was off duty.

Some funny things happened while we were in the cottage. One day our second daughter appeared in the kitchen with a bunch of flowers, which she smilingly presented to her grandmother.

'Thank you, my darling. Where did you get those lovely flowers?'

Catherine was not telling. It later transpired that she had crawled under the churchyard gate, just opposite the house, where she had found lots of pretty flowers. So she had brought a great collection of them to her granny. Little dear.

On another occasion, I found time to plant a considerable row of salvias in the new flowerbed skirting the drive. Catherine chattered away beside me the whole time. The trays empty, my back aching, I straightened up – only the last two salvias were in the bed, the others had all been tweaked out and dropped on the drive. Little dear.

Almost opposite our cottage, looking the other way from the churchyard, there was what had been the coachhouse to a sizeable property. It was inhabited by a rather unsavoury chap who, amongst other things, kept goats for milking. At this time we had a lovely little black Labrador puppy – well, sort of teenager. One day the goat-keeper rang up in high dudgeon – would we please keep our bloody dog under control? It was a ruddy nuisance. When Mary enquired what the pup was doing, she discovered that Judy had been visiting the goats and milking them. She apparently found goat's milk very tasty.

Old Jacob and his wife lingered on in their big old house for a number of years after he eventually retired. Childless, they were both in their eighties, and they positively rattled in a house of four reception rooms and eight bedrooms, not to mention an enormous kitchen and two sculleries. They had lived there since the day of their marriage. It was Jacob who suggested that we consider moving in with them, to live entirely separately but with Mary looking after the household affairs. It was agreed that, in the event of Jacob dying first, the old lady would go into a home of some sort, and that we would buy the property then – at probate valuation. With some misgivings we moved. We did not sell the cottage immediately, in case the arrangement proved too difficult. We rented it out, which we later discovered was not a good idea at all. Our tenants did considerable damage and stole a rather charming watercolour of the village church, which we never recovered.

One of the first things I did on moving was to ask the GPO to install a new telephone in the big house, with the same number we had at the cottage. This would avoid any confusion which might arise from patients having to get accustomed to a new number. The GPO maintained that this was impossible – because the big house was already served by a line from a different local exchange on the far side of the main road. This would complicate maintenance, they said. I was fortunate in having been supervisor of a military exchange in 1940, under the command of the formidable General Montgomery. When I pointed out that the maintenance crew for either small exchange came from the same place and must approach up the same road, the GPO agreed that I should retain my old number. It had a delightfully rural ring to it – Woolley 319 – and yes, as well as there being a hamlet of Woolley, most of the local farmers kept a few sheep.

There was plenty of room for us to enjoy a good measure of privacy. The old folk had Jacob's big study, a big bedroom, a spare room and their own bathroom, while we had the rest. Mary took them their meals in the study. But life at the big house was not wholly straightforward. Old Jacob had not long since broken his arm in a fall inspecting a local water tower. He had insisted on not going to hospital, saying that he could treat the limb at home just as well. A few weeks after the accident I found him standing on a ladder in the garden, sawing a big branch off an apple tree.

'Jacob, what on earth are you doing? You really should not be using that saw.'

'Just a little pruning. Someone's got to do it. Yes, I suppose it does hurt a bit.'

Sadly it was not very long after we moved in that the old boy died. Nothing to do with pruning the apple tree. In due course, Janet moved out and we bought the house – including three garages and the two and a half acres of garden – for three thousand three hundred pounds. Yes, we sold the cottage at the same time, although it did not quite pay for the house. Not long after this I made an interesting discovery. Although Jacob and his father-in-law had between them held the post of Medical Officer of Health for the Rural District for sixty-seven years (Jacob's successor lasting no more than six months,) the downstairs WC had no seal at all between the pan and the pipe.

I could have stayed there for ever. There was but one thing wrong with it – its isolation. The family was growing, and it seemed unfair that the children should be cut off from their friends – unless Mary took them and fetched them in the car they might just as well have been on a desert island. And this made immense demands upon her, too. I was very reluctant to move, but it was the right thing to do. We sold that lovely house for eleven thousand pounds and bought a comfortable Victorian house in 'my' main village, not a hundred yards from the surgery I had built a few years before. Across the yard was a large barn that had been a granary, which was to prove very useful later. Once more we had bought more land than we needed, so I sold off an acre or so for building, which was some recompense to me for having to give up the old house and went towards several improvements. At least we were comfortable, and the children were within walking or cycling distance of most things. The scene was set for a further series of excitements.

Harry was a fairly near neighbour. He had a biggish farm adjoining the village. His two sons farmed with him but had their own homes and families, one daughter was married, the other still lived at home. Harry and his wife, Sheila, would have rattled a bit in the big farmhouse, had it not been for Sheila's ninety-year-old father. He was a funny old man, unhappily rapidly losing his grip on life. One morning Harry asked me to call to see him. He was in bed and making an awful fuss – poor Sheila just did not know what to do with him. I went up to the old chap's bedroom. He did not take very kindly to my visit, insisting that his room was full of sheep. Nothing I said would persuade him otherwise. He was becoming something of a handful and akin to my later trials with the drug addict in London. My rescuer this time was not a lithe and lissome lass – it was all sixteen and a half stone of Harry. He soon came stomping in.

'What's the matter, then, Granddad? Is it them woollies again? Don't you worry, I'll deal with them all right.'

With that Harry whacked his hefty walking stick on the old man's brass bedrail again and again, shouting and swearing at the illusory sheep, before stomping off down the landing, his voice receding. After a short pause Harry returned to the bedroom. If it had been possible for someone of his size, he almost tip-toed in.

'It's all right, Granddad. Them bloody sheep's all penned up safe. They'll be no more trouble now.'

The old man closed his eyes and went to sleep. Another lesson learned.

It was Harry's turn to be sick. He had had increasing pain and stiffness in one hip for a long time, which he had tried to ignore. When he at last acknowledged that he needed help, he was very reluctant to accept my suggestion that he might do best with a hip replacement. He didn't want that sort of thing. I thought of a way I might win him over.

'Harry, I tell you what. You're a Mason, aren't you? A very good friend of mine is a Mason – he also happens to be a rather distinguished orthopaedic surgeon in London. He's doing a lot of hips. Why don't you go and see him? See what he has to offer? You've no need to say yes – but he is something of an authority.'

That was acceptable. Harry very soon went off to London to see Geoffrey. The following day I decided to call at the farm at the beginning of my 'safari' – his car was by the front door, so he was probably in.

'Hello, Harry. How did you get on with my friend Geoffrey?'

'He's a damned nice fellow, that 'e is. No operation until I've lost three stone. Then 'e says 'e'll do me, and I shall run a marathon. I've started my diet already – not a drop of whisky till I've made it to thirteen stone odd.'

It was only a couple of months or so before Harry had lost his surplus and had a brand new hip. I went to see him the day after he got home. He was sitting in the living room, reading the *Farmers' Weekly*.

'Well doctor, you were bloody right. You'll have a scotch. I know you don't drink at this time of day, but this is different. We've got something to celebrate. And you like to spoil it with water, I know. And I can have one too, now I've 'ad the bloody thing done. You pour, doctor – you know where the cupboard is.'

With that he jumped out of his very low chair and almost ran along the long stone passage to the kitchen to get me some water. He had left his stick by his chair, and he maintained that it was for prodding the cattle only. A not entirely sobering thought was that he once told me he customarily bought a case of whisky each fortnight.

One of the highlights of living in this village house of ours was to do with our Jack Russell terrier. 'Little Henry' had succeeded Judy. He was quite a character. He was not content with chasing cats up trees or attacking passing Land Rovers' front wheels. When they built a row of eight small shops just up the road, he took it as his duty to parade up and down them each morning and select his shop of the day. Then he would sit outside and decide which potential customer was allowed into the shop and which was not. This was not wholly popular with the poor traders, who made their displeasure quite clear. I spoke to 'Little Henry' sternly. I have no idea whether he understood me or not, but he certainly changed his tactics. Instead of the shops, he chose to station himself outside the surgery, where he assumed the same duties – deciding which patients might enter. Free access, my foot. Sadly, 'Little Henry' had to go.

An unusual feature of our sojourn in that house was that on a mad impulse I bought an old Royal Navy Seaplane tender, which spent many months on chocks in the front garden, while I renovated her. She was lovely – all forty foot of her. With oak frames and double diagonal mahogany planking, she really was a thing of beauty. I had the two seven-and-a-half-litre Perkins engines repaired and I enlisted the aid of a patient in the giant task of dealing with the carpentry. This included the building of safety rails from scratch, as she had had none in her heyday. Ben and I spent as much time as we could spare on this task – the same age as me, he had spent his war service in the Royal Navy. We modified her so as to reduce the size of the open well to provide a two-berth cabin aft of the wheelhouse, which left us with just enough room for a couple of rather odd-shaped bunks in the 'sharp end'. The dream was that we would be able to go to France on holiday. Yes, down to the Wash by river, and then round the coast and across. Slowly all took shape. I even did a postal course in coastal navigation.

One Saturday I was clearing up in the surgery, relishing the prospect of the hundred-yard walk to get on with the boat, when there was a knock on the door. Damn, I thought I was finished. I opened the door to find a rather scruffy small boy smiling up at me. I recognised him straight away.

'Well, what can I do for you, Archie?'

'Doctor, will you do my laces up for me? Please?'

Of course, I could not refuse. Archie probably made a bob or two out of that caper. His pals must have dared him to do it.

For reasons I shall make clear in the next chapter, we decided to move on again. Realising at school that I might not be able to go in for medicine (because of the cost) I had always known that my second choice of career would be architecture. At least you got paid for learning in that theatre – there was much to be said for the system of apprenticeship. Soon I was to fulfil one of my earliest ambitions. We found a beautiful plot of land, sloping down to the river and with an unspoilt view across green fields as far as the eye could see. It was a lovely spot. And what a challenge to design a house that fitted into the slope. And I was not a total amateur either – after all I had designed the surgery myself. But this was different – this was to be something quite special. We would be able to tie up the boat at the bottom of the garden. If we could cut a small chunk out of the river bank, we would have our own tiny port.

We spent weeks planning that house, starting before we actually bought the land – and before we had applied for planning permission. There was no harm in planning. And, better still, I had a patient who was an architect. At least he could draw better plans than I could, and he could deal with the Planning Authority more effectively, too. So Robert was dragged into the business. We included a substantial solar heating unit with a very sophisticated control system – the pump even came on once on Christmas Day. We also built a massive tank just below the house, to act as storage for roof-water and as reservoir for some heat exchange units. This was to be something special. Distinctly environmentally friendly.

Our chosen builder was not a patient of mine, but he had been highly recommended by Robert – who ought to know something about the local tradesmen. His ageing 'bricky' George, whose last job this was before retiring, wasn't my patient either. But the plumber was a patient of Maurice's – and a damned good plumber too, who specialised in solar heating. The planners were a bit of a pain. Initially they insisted on our installing 'perpendicular' windows in our brand new modern house, to tie in with the church architecture of the region. It was a ludicrous demand – happily abandoned after I pointed out that the house would be almost completely hidden from the public gaze and that there was not a solitary perpendicular window to be seen from the site either.

As the topping out approached, our eldest daughter brought her husband to us on a few days' visit. Of course, what better than to ask him to do the topping out? It was only after he had obliged that we discovered he was scared stiff of heights. Dear Bill, he did it to please us. At last we moved in. And then the matter of making a garden became a serious priority.

I never saw patients at this house. By the time we moved in I was working almost exclusively in London. But for a very short time we did have one resident patient – my very dear father-in-law. Doctor Spears could not have been kinder to the old chap, and he died very peacefully, in his nineties. Happily, I only had to ask the good doctor to see me once in the years we were there.

My most vivid recollection of that house has nothing to do with patients. Mary was away doing the granny act, helping our eldest daughter and her family, and I was all alone in the house. One morning I got up rather early and walked out onto the long balcony overlooking the river. Down at the bottom of the garden, just yards from our lovely boat, there was a swan's nest which I had been observing for some days. The process of hatching was under way. Today the cob had gone off up the river, leaving his mate sitting on the eggs. Suddenly I saw a great grey heron swoop down over the nest, squawking aggressively, flying on to perch in a tree on the bank beyond. No sooner had it settled than a second heron did the same from the other direction. I stood transfixed, as the two birds made integrated attacks, obviously trying to get the pen off the nest. Each time the lovely bird stood up, lashing out wildly at the herons with wings and beak – but she did not leave the nest. These birds did four or five sweeps each until the cob came back then they flew off in defeat. I had no idea that herons indulged in teamwork. I was shivering with cold and I might be late for work. It had certainly been worth it, but how I wished I had had a camera at the ready.

We spent some happy years in our dream house. Perhaps the biggest problem was that I was seldom there. In spite of having abandoned general practice in order to reduce my workload, that load seemed to mount relentlessly. And I spent far too much time driving up and down to London – not only a waste of time, but an awful waste of money and pretty wearing. It seemed only sense for us to move to where most of the work was. Yes, we sold that house and moved once more.

This time we bought the lease of a flat in the West End. It was two minutes' walk to my consulting room (rather than the nearly two hours it took to drive). It was not much more to Oxford Street, and everything was at our fingertips. Museums, galleries and all the magic of London were ours to grasp. Mary was ecstatic about our move. While I agreed that it made sense, I could never forget my attachment to the countryside – and to country people. But once again our new abode brought us some new laughs.

Mrs Cousins lived almost next door to the Royal Albert Hall. Recently widowed, her dear companion was an ageing dachshund. Rupert developed paralysis of both hind legs and, gutsy little fellow that he was, he eventually rubbed the skin off his 'knees' by running along with his front legs, dragging his paralysed hind legs along the ground. Mrs Cousins took Rupert to the vet. His advice was that the dog should be put down. Disc protrusion – the cause of the paralysis – was a common ailment in dachshunds, and sadly incurable. In some pique Mrs Cousins took Rupert to another vet. No, there really was nothing that could be done for the poor little chap – he would have to go. Mrs Cousins would have none of it. Twice a day she would carry Rupert to Kensington Gardens. There she would put him down and hold his tail, so that he might run about with his front legs, while not scraping the skin off his hind legs.

The surprising outcome of her noble action was twofold. Lifting Rupert's tail put his spine into extension, while his front legs applied traction as he charged ahead. In a week or two his paralysis had totally vanished. Nonetheless he died soon after. However, stooping for prolonged periods as she made her way through Kensington Gardens with some loss of dignity ensured that Mrs Cousins developed an agonising pain in her back, which is how I came to meet her. I got rid of her pain all right – but I very much doubt whether I would have succeeded if Rupert had still been around.

Since schooldays I had always loved singing. I did not do it very well, but I enjoyed it very much. But what has this to do with living in the West End? Towards the end of a long day I welcomed my last patient, Mr Kurtz. Perhaps in his early seventies, he ran his own jewellery manufacturing business in London. For some reason I asked him where he came from. He told me that he originated from Prague, adding that he was in Vienna shortly before the war had broken out, but that he had spent almost all of the war in the RAF, as a fighter pilot.

'Mr Kurtz, what on earth were you doing in Vienna?'

'Oh, I was an opera singer. When Hitler walked in I walked out – and joined the RAF.'

'I bet your favourite language for singing is Italian – with German a good second.'

'Oh, yes indeed.'

'Do you know the lovely song, "*Rosen brach ich nachts Dir am dunklen Hage*"?'

'Of course. It is a delight.'

At this the consulting room was filled with song, as we sang an unpremeditated duet. I wished my voice had matched his. What everybody else in the house thought I did not know. I did not bother, either. It was such a lovely, spontaneous episode.

David and Angela were an interesting couple. He was first of the two to come under my care. A concert pianist turned conductor, he had a postural problem which required sorting out. This was not very difficult to overcome. Angela was next on my list. She had a painful neck which she found very tiresome. I thought I had dealt with her satisfactorily, when she rang to ask me to come to the house – she was in a lot of pain again. They lived in a splendid modern house in north London, which sported a very handsome open staircase. It so happened that I was to drive with Mary almost past the door that evening to attend a meeting of the debating society I had founded so many years before, so I called on my way. I was able to help Angela a great deal, but before I left I was asked to see David as well. The 'while you're here doctor' syndrome again. David wanted advice about the height of his piano stool. He demonstrated his problem. I stood far too long listening in rapture to the lovely sounds coming from his gorgeous grand piano. Then, remembering that Mary was in the car, I gave my advice, excused myself and fled.

Some time later we were invited to dinner with them. They had just become grandparents and asked us to join them in celebration. Always with an ear for dialects, I could not restrain myself.

'Do tell me, Angela, am I not right in saying your roots are not far from Bradford?'

Her grandmother had come from Rotherham! The evening became even more relaxed. She then told us a delightful story regarding an old friend of theirs. Tied up in the world of music, Jordan lived in South Africa. Whenever he visited London, they used to meet. There came the day when he had arranged to lunch with Angela and David. He rang mid-morning to say he would be late. At about one the doorbell rang. Angela came dashing downstairs, anticipating a jolly reunion and not knowing that David was almost by the door. As she descended the lovely staircase, she saw through the open doorway first a pair of feet, then a briefcase.

'Eh, Jordan, tha daft bugger.'

It was only one or two seconds later that she got far enough down the stairs to see the rest of their visitor – it was the piano tuner.

Was our West End flat to be the end of our wanderings? No. Ultimately I retired from clinical practice and we moved to France. But more of that later.

9

Role Reversal

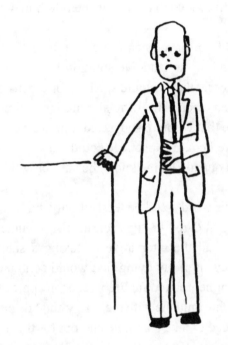

I got away with it pretty well for a good many years, but I suppose I did rather ask for it. As I mentioned earlier, I discovered that I had a dangerously high blood pressure – and I retired from general practice. This decision was to provoke a rare mix of laughter and tears – certainly things did not go entirely smoothly. First I talked to Mary about it – she was a bit alarmed at the whole matter, but she accepted that this was probably the best way out. It seemed worth a try. I also discussed the question with Maurice and Dick, although by then we had gone our separate ways, each of us needing to take in a new partner as the practice populations grew. They were both a bit shocked at the actual pressure recorded and agreed that retirement from general practice would offer a reasonable chance for me to avoid early disaster. So I went to see the Clerk to the Executive Council (as it was then) to find out just where I stood

Lloyd Thomas could not have been more helpful. I first told him of the problem, and of the tentative solution I had come up with. I next asked him whether I would qualify for a pension at my age, as I had not then reached the official minimum retirement age. He was pretty sure that I would, so I asked him to give me an idea of the sort of figure I could expect. He could not answer this, but volunteered to find out and let me know the answer within the week.

He was as good as his word – and better. Not only did he come up with a figure I had not dared to hope for, he also volunteered the information that I had the alternative of taking a standard pension, which in the event of my dying first would continue for Mary at fifty per cent for her remaining lifetime, or an appreciably increased pension which would die with me. Mary and I discussed this at length and decided to take a gamble and opt for the higher level. So I told my new practice partner of my decision and we agreed a date for her to take over – the end of June. She appeared perfectly happy with that arrangement. On that basis I formally resigned, requesting a pension 'suitably reduced by my not yet having reached minimum retirement age'. All seemed set for a tranquil withdrawal from at least some of the mad rush. With reasonable luck I should escape an early stroke.

Tranquillity was far from what I achieved. I was due to hand over everything on a Tuesday. During the afternoon of the Friday before, I had a phone call from Maurice, suggesting I ring a Dr Clarke at the Ministry of Health. There appeared to be some doubt as to my eligibility for a pension at all. I could not think why it was that Maurice had become involved in the matter – and neither could he. Anyway, he gave me the number to ring, suggesting that I should not delay. Dr Clarke was not yet back from lunch – it was about three-thirty in the afternoon. I asked his secretary if she would be kind enough to ask him to ring me back as soon as he returned to his office – as a matter of some urgency. I am pretty sure my blood pressure went up alarmingly, but I dared not take it. Nothing happened, either to the telephone or to me.

Happily, Dr Clarke's home telephone number was given in the Medical Directory. I rang him that evening in near desperation. A rather odd voice asked me my name (I had given it already) before assuring me that Dr Clarke was having dinner with me. I just could not persuade her that this was not the case. I was pretty sure the owner of the voice was distinctly tipsy. There was no point in continuing the conversation. By Saturday morning I was frantic. I rang again. This time it was Dr Clarke who answered. Apologising for bothering him at home, I told him my problem – in three days' time I should be virtually without income. His reply was casual in the extreme.

'Oh, I'm so sorry. Dr Paterson, yes I remember. There seems to have been something of a query in your case – a matter as to whether or not you are retiring on the grounds of ill-health. You will need to have a medical examination, but I'm afraid the local examiner for your area has just retired, and we have not yet replaced him.'

'Dr Clarke, you have had my case under consideration for a number of months. Most of my income ceases next week. I can get to your home in not much more than a couple of hours – perhaps you could check me out yourself?'

'Oh, I can't do that, I'm afraid. I'm playing golf at eleven.'

I probably got even nearer to a stroke at that. Three weeks later I was seen by a very pleasant doctor in the next county, who heartily agreed that I should be out. At length the mystery was resolved. Some bright spark at the Ministry of Health had come up with the proposition that my resignation was on the grounds of ill-health – though I had made no mention of this in my application. The end result was that my pension was to be increased to what it would have been if I had done a further six years in the service. After the agonies of indecision, this was good news indeed.

In theory, the threat of serious stroke should have been markedly reduced by my decision. Was it hell! The Monday after my fraught discussion with Dr Clarke brought a further shock. When I brought up the matter, my practice partner firmly announced that she would not buy the surgery I had built twenty years previously. But this was in our partnership agreement – no question. It was then that I realised I had made a serious error of judgement when taking her into partnership a few years back. I had thought she was just administratively a bit waffly, although she was obviously very bright as a doctor. She had never actually signed the partnership agreement. I told her that I must sell the property as, with a sharp decline in income, I needed the capital. If she did not want to buy it, then she would have to find other premises, so that I could relieve myself of an unacceptable burden. She flatly declined to move out. When I suggested she pay a rent, she again refused point-blank. Why I did not explode at that I cannot say. It certainly did no good to my blood pressure. And it was eight months before I had a penny rent – and then only on the threat of legal action. The following February she finally moved out, allowing me to sell the property.

It may be hard to believe, but this was not the end of my woes. Over the previous twenty-five years I had assiduously put by the odd bob or two. Being a dunce at finance, I had entrusted almost all my life savings to a patient, who happened to make his living as a financial advisor. Tony Lever was very bright – too bright. Not long after the horrid business with my practice partner he played the financial fiddle act. I lost almost all my life savings. I was warned too late by a colleague who had retrieved his savings in the nick of time. Tony went to court, was found guilty, fined a ludicrously small sum and told not to be a naughty boy again. Only one of the several others he had cheated got a penny back. Not very good for a dodgy blood pressure! In spite of this I slowly settled down, as I resumed a rather more placid life. But I did need to take some medication.

Then I experienced something new. I developed a troublesome pain in my tummy. Nothing much, really, but it just did not go away. I mentioned this to my friend, Dr Spears. To be on the safe side he sent me for a barium enema. This was not to prove my favourite experience, and I doubt whether Ewart found it much fun either. It seemed as if about three gallons of the horrid stuff was pumped into me – not a comfortable business. When it was all over the very efficient nurse told me to go off to the loo to get rid of the barium. I sat for some unrewarding minutes, to nil effect. Then I realised why my journey was fruitless – I had had an intravenous injection of a muscle relaxant before the X-ray and now my gut muscle had been effectively put out of action. Giving up the unequal struggle, I collected my very beautiful X-rays and waddled to my car. I drove home in some discomfort, unable to do up my trousers. Looking at the X-rays, I thought the multiple diverticuli of my colon were quite pretty – thankfully they did not matter at all. I suppose it was worth it to get a definitive answer as to what the problem was.

After lunch one Sunday at my sister's house I was chasing a four-year-old granddaughter round the garden. It had rained a little that morning. Cornering too fast, I slipped on the damp grass and fell, hitting my head on a rock at the side of the fish-pool. There was blood everywhere. My sister's doctor was out on a visit. Giving me a replacement for my sodden handkerchief, she insisted that she drive me the ten miles into Casualty. That was a horrifying journey – she was in a hurry, and her style of driving was not like mine. I was terrified. The pleasant young houseman in Casualty put in seven very tidy small stitches – and all the while he insisted on calling me 'Sir'. He must have thought I looked very old. The journey back was a little more tranquil, but it was relaxing for me to drive myself home after that somewhat traumatic weekend.

That was to be my last experience of British medicine for a good many years. Not long after this we moved to France. With plenty to keep me out of mischief, I intended to forget about being a patient. Of course, I was wrong again. Slowly my left hip became more and more stiff and painful. My delightful new doctor, Pierre Bonnet, was a gentle and quiet man who invariably ushered his patient out to the front door of the surgery before inviting his next one to precede him down the corridor to his consulting room. I thought this was a good start. He had a computer on his desk, and produced any necessary letter of referral on the spot (with a copy for me) as well as any prescription. This time he shook his head – there was nothing but a hip replacement for me. He referred me to a very remarkable professor an hour's drive away.

Within the week I was sitting in Alain Gauthier's palatial

consulting room. It seemed to me a little odd, but its walls were lined with photographs of wartime military aircraft – some of which I thought I recognised. In particular there were pictures of both the Wellesley and the Wellington bombers. The atmosphere was very relaxed, and I felt I really must ask him why he had these lovely pictures on his walls.

'Professor Gauthier, tell me why it is that you have these remarkable photographs in your consulting room?'

'My dear colleague, that is easy to answer. I have to admit to you that I was for a while undecided as to whether to read medicine or aeronautical engineering. When I took the plunge into medicine, I looked for the most challenging arena – for a would-be engineer. I chose joint replacement. Now I do nothing but hips and knees.'

'Of course, you must know the name of Barnes Wallis.'

'Indeed I do. He was an absolute genius.'

'I must tell you something, Professor. In 1939, as a first-year medical student, I sat through a lecture by him on his wonderful innovation of geodetic construction. I shall never forget his little model, made of two discs of wood joined by double helices of 18-gauge copper wire. You could distort the wires in or out with your little finger, but the discs could not be twisted, and he eventually stood on the up-ended contraption. It was he who designed the frames of both the Wellington and the Wellesley bombers.'

'What a fascinating experience. I think I understand your interest. Now I have to introduce you to another engineering novelty – custom-built prostheses for the individual patient, designed, milled and polished by computer – truly made to measure. That is what I propose for you.'

When he had finished his clinical examination Professor Gauthier really surprised me. He told me that he insisted on a month's programme of preparation for the operation, including the giving of blood four weeks running (so that it would be available to me as required, with no risk of mismatching). When would I like to have the operation?

I delayed it by a few weeks, as I was due to teach in England very soon. The whole set-up was inspiring. The simple idea of having one's own blood available at operation was so obviously good. Francois Gère, the anaesthetist, decided that he would give me an epidural. Like a chump, I imagined that I would be conscious during the operation. After my pre-medical injection I was wheeled down to the operating theatre, where I was met by a very comely nurse, who bulged in all the right places. Sitting on the side of the theatre trolley, I scarcely felt the needle go in – the last thing I remembered was falling forwards, my head coming to rest in her ample bosom. I woke up in my bed, with a new hip. The result was magic. I was weight-bearing on the second post-operative day and on the ninth day I walked up and down stairs under the supervision of an excellent physiotherapist – and went home.

And then I nearly spoilt it. At my first follow-up consultation I was seen by Professor Gauthier's charming assistant, Dr Carole Lange. Pretty pleased with what she saw, she leaned on my knee as I lay on the couch and asked me to lift my leg against resistance. Perhaps too pleased with myself, I did as I was told rather vigorously. There was an audible snap and I was in absolute agony. There followed a mad dash in a wheelchair to the X-ray department – I must have broken my femur just where the prosthesis had been installed. The whole exercise would prove to have been in vain. Happily it was nothing worse than pulling off a small osteophyte. I went home in some discomfort but greatly relieved. And I have had not a solitary twinge in the subsequent thirteen years.

A couple of years later I experienced crippling pain across my shoulders and up into my neck. Pierre Bonnet agreed with me that this must be polymyalgia rheumatica. With my instant prescription I bore away my letter of introduction to Professor Claude Weygand. Gosh this was efficient. And yes, I saw him within days. He politely pooh-poohed my diagnosis, but on examining me he suddenly excused himself and left the examination room at speed. Mary was sitting next door in the consulting room. She had no idea where he had gone – or why. It was about five minutes later that he returned – with the Professor of Cardiology, Anton Brun. Mary went home without me – I was admitted on the spot. Sure enough, it was my long-standing high blood pressure that had finally put things out of kilter. After that I spent years going to and from the hospital, sometimes spending a night or two there. I used to call that hospital my '*maison secondaire*'.

The evening of one of my earlier stays there brought something of a surprise. It must have been close on seven o'clock and I was wondering when Mary would ring me when Professor Brun walked in. This was his last visit of the day, and he chatted away for a while. He seemed to be in no hurry – and, amongst other topics, we happily discussed the beneficial effect of red wine on the coronary arteries. He went into some detail on this subject, and I found his comments extremely interesting. Then I asked him his views about whisky as a painkiller. He agreed that its beneficial effects had been conclusively proved. And he was delighted to learn that I had been involved in producing some of early the evidence, when a final-year medical student.

'Do you care for whisky yourself, Professor?'

'As a matter of fact I do. Perhaps, as a Frenchman, I should not admit that in public.'

'Ah, but this is private. As a further matter of fact, I have a bottle in my locker – and I have a spare glass. Would you care to join me?'

And there we were, Professor Brun sitting on the side of my hospital bed, enjoying a not too modest scotch apiece, when Mary rang. I remembered the grateful Mr Tonkin experimenting on me long ago. This time it was a single malt – Laphroaig.

In spite of Professor Brun's noble efforts, and in spite of my dutifully taking a sensible dose of wine and whisky each day, my wretched engine room remained in some turmoil. It just would not operate smoothly. Eventually I had a pacemaker installed. Everything went ominously well. I was fascinated to watch a television screen and see the thing being put in place. These chaps really did seem to know what they were doing. And it worked like a charm. My wretched heart settled to a proper rhythm – for the first time in ages.

A week after its installation Mary and I flew to Toronto to visit our eldest daughter. I remembered not to go through the screening device at customs, instead being frisked by a very jolly fellow. All went well as we roared over the Atlantic, until we were informed that the plane was being diverted to Halifax. No reason for this was given. We disembarked, collected our baggage and went through customs and thence to the departures lounge. There were no seats available in the overcrowded lounge and we had to stand in a queue for more than twenty minutes – waiting to re-board the very plane we had come in on. We even sat in the same seats. I was not feeling at all well. We made it to Toronto by midnight, to be met by an anxious daughter, and I was very glad to get to bed within the hour.

I awoke on Sunday morning in frank heart failure. Our daughter was unable to contact her doctor. After breakfast she and

I walked very slowly to the nearby pharmacy. Mr Keen could not have been more helpful – not only did he find me a chair to sit on, he gave me a small supply of a drug which would tide me over until I could see the doctor. All was well in a few days. Or was it? I managed to leave my pacemaker identification card in my shirt pocket. The washing machine pulled it out of the pocket, took the document out of its little plastic envelope and chewed up all the precious details – it left only the front fold with my name and address. On my return, Professor Brun laughed long and loud – but suggested I should not repeat the process. Three years later I was to run out of one of my drugs in Toronto – and the good Mr Keen rescued me once more.

My eyesight has never been really good. I remember having to wear glasses all day at the age of eleven. But I grew to accept specs as necessary, and I was fortunate to have only the one serious episode of losing them recalled earlier, during my days in Casualty. I had tried contact lenses when I was about fifty, but it was a bit late in the day – I was near to needing bifocals. It was when I started seeing double that I got worried. It only happened intermittently, but there was no warning. The vital question had to be, which of two oncoming cars to avoid? Time for another decision. I had no option but to give up driving. This was a real wrench. I had relied on being self-propelled for so long. I used to do twenty-five to thirty thousand miles a year in rural practice, and I had driven in eight European countries, as well as in India and Burma. With real sadness, I sold my forty-sixth car. With even a loaf of bread out of reach, we had to make yet another move.

I was finding the walk uphill from the shops more and more of a struggle. So we moved again and found ourselves somewhere more or less on the level. This must be all right, I certainly thought so. Of course I was wrong again. This time there was no warning.

One evening I just lost consciousness and fell to the floor for no apparent reason. Mary was very concerned, but I soon got up – although I had no recollection of the episode at all. What on earth was she fussing about? Perhaps I could have ignored it. In fact, I rather think I did for a start. But weeks later I did it again. And again. These were true 'drop attacks,' and all the numerous investigations instigated by Dr Ventoux revealed nothing. There was therefore nothing to be done. My sixth attack occurred while Mary was ill in bed – I collapsed on the bedroom floor, hitting my head on the corner of my bedside table as I fell. Happily we were not alone at the time, and the good Dr Ventoux had to mend my bloody scalp at bedtime – once again I remembered nothing about the fall, wondering why I woke up in the morning with blood on my pillow and a dressing on my head.

I had recently had a replacement of my excellent pacemaker. The original one had served me well for eight years. It was a long time since I qualified as a doctor. Now I really believed I had attained professional patienthood, but I know which role I prefer. So what next?

The next trial was for me to develop pins and needles and pain in my left hand. It must arise in my ageing neck. Scans revealed a pretty worn-out spine – too bad. No, the next loss of dignity was not a drop attack. I just tripped. I fell down a flight of four steps, hitting my head on a wooden post and crashing onto a concrete floor on both knees. Thank heavens there was someone else in the house as I could not have got up unaided. I was devastated when, not long after that, Mary died. And yes, I tripped on uneven paving and fell again – this time breaking a bone in my right hand. Surely this was enough?

My return to England seemed sensible. In practice it was not very funny, although the family were quite wonderful in their help

140

– on both sides of the Channel. I settled into my new home. I could scarcely believe it – my hand then got worse a similar problem arose in my feet, and I developed pain and stiffness in my wonderful hip. It would be six months before I was finally able to discuss what might be done for me. Should I have come back from France? It really is more fun being a doctor.

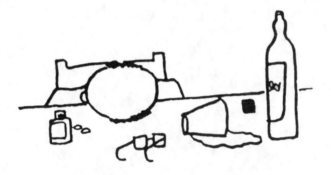

10

What is All This Rot About Retirement?

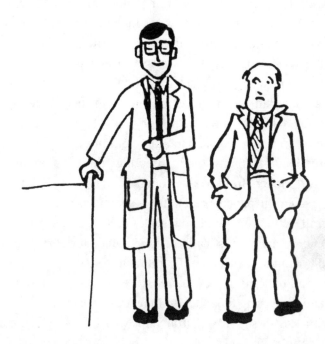

As described earlier, my first retirement was indeed a trifle traumatic. What with inefficiency on the part of the Department of Health, a somewhat devious partner and a criminal financial advisor, Lloyd Thomas's stalwart efforts on my behalf came near to being nullified. However, in the end we triumphed. Now I would have ample time to pursue my chosen interests, without resort to over-drive. That was the plan. At first it seemed to work.

But bit by bit my days got shorter, filled nearer to the brim with every new task.

In spite of a modest growth in clinical work, I was now free to devote myself more rigorously to teaching. That meant planning courses, advertising their availability, booking places for participants, arranging venues, as well as the simple business side of things. It also involved attending meetings all over the place, meeting more people who shared my interests – from all over Europe, and beyond. It demanded more writing, with further publishing in collaboration with Leonard Brown as well as on my own. For good measure I also acted as Honorary Secretary to one national association for eight years, following this by being its President for a further three years. On top of that I served as Chairman of an international scientific committee for five years, which involved planning and directing three international seminars for teachers from twelve countries.

Writing scientific papers is great fun – so long as you do not fall into the trap of thinking you know best. Of course, first you must ensure that you have statistically valid evidence for what you say is the truth. But the real secret of producing a sound paper lies in thinking of all the criticisms you are likely to provoke before you write it, and answering them before they are put. This leaves your critics with less to say. My patron saint was Doubting Thomas, and he seldom let me down in something like one hundred papers, most of them written after my first retirement. One such occasion stands out in my mind. I had spoken about a subject in which there remained substantial disagreement within the medical profession. I had been very careful to distinguish between proven fact and reasonable supposition, stressing that we are often uncertain of particular matters, and that honesty is the best policy. There were two rather bright doctors at this particular meeting. Suddenly they spoke up – while I was still speaking – chanting, 'We don't know. We just don't know.'

The whole audience fell about laughing, and it became the theme for the rest of the meeting – repeated on numerous occasions. Not much later I published a paper entitled 'I can tell – an impediment to progress'. I thought there were too many 'I can tell' merchants around. I rather think the paper was not greatly appreciated by some. Retirement was certainly not proving to be boring.

This was all simple stuff. One of the things I found a real challenge was the international congress we hosted in London. In doing this I encountered some rather difficult problems. Because of the scale of the undertaking, we agreed to engage a firm of conference organisers to deal with the background chores of setting it all up, arranging venues and catering. We also agreed that one member of our committee should seek financial backing – he had previous experience of doing this very successfully for another association. As the time of the congress approached, we realised that we had nothing firm in the way of financial support. At one committee meeting in mid-planning stage he was asked what progress he was making over finance.

'None, really. I've been far too busy with my practice. Actually I haven't asked anybody yet.'

The threat of a stroke loomed once again! How I refrained from doing that man grievous bodily harm I do not know. Indeed, at the last moment it was I who secured the only financial backing we got for the whole congress – from a trades union. By the time the congress opened I had written no fewer than eight hundred letters. And, for good measure, Leonard and I edited a book of fifty-five of the papers presented at it. This was rapidly followed by our definitive text. In spite of the sponsorship setback, on the whole the occupational therapy of retirement was working well for me.

The congress over, it was time for me to retire – for the second time. I gave up clinical work, although I continued to teach with Leonard for some years to come. This must surely herald the beginning of loafing about with little to do. Was it hell! I mentioned earlier that we moved to France – this was shortly after the London congress. There was a story behind this. Some while earlier we had mounted a sort of rescue operation for one of our daughters, then working in southern France. We had asked her to find somewhere big enough to divide into two, so that she could have a permanent home and the rest of the family might share a holiday retreat. She had found one which sounded ideal, and we had booked our tickets to go over to sign the necessary documents. Two days before we were due to go, a very distressed daughter had rung to tell us we had been gazumped.

'OK then. We've got our air tickets, and we are not wasting them. Find somewhere else in the meantime and we'll go ahead with an alternative over the weekend.'

What we had eventually bought was not big enough for what we had anticipated – but the rescue operation took precedence over dreams of holidays in the sunshine. We had bought a pleasant little cottage in a remote hamlet, within easy driving distance of some lovely spots. The crisis was over. Months later we had been visiting when the farmer who had sold us the cottage offered us the small barn next door – for conversion into a house. It was pretty hideous, made of ugly concrete blocks, though it had quite an attractive gently sloping tiled roof. Mary was very discouraged by it. The more I looked at it, the more was I convinced that it could be made more than adequate. A plain oblong building, about thirty-four feet by twenty-six, with one large door and one high window onto the road. It certainly did seem a bit dreary from the outside.

It was going inside and looking up which persuaded me – there was a massive beam across the full width of the barn, five or six inches thick and more than a foot deep. From the centre of this beam there arose a king-post to the ridge, supported by a splay of four oblique timbers, two to the ridge and the other two to the upper of two purlins on either side. It was this splay of timber work which I found so delightful. Surely we could retain those lovely timbers and cover up all the nastiness. In the end we had bought the ugly place.

In the last two years before my second retirement Mary and I took a small caravan down there for two or three weeks at a time, several times a year. We took a different route each time, really enjoying avoiding the mad rush of motorways. The beautiful beam had sagged a bit, leaving a one and a half inch gap between it and the king-post's seating. Some chump had applied a steel loop over this defect, which had the effect of the beam being supported by the king-post, rather than the other way round. My first job was to correct this fault. I took two stout timbers just too long to fit under the middle of the beam, their feet jammed on the concrete floor about two feet apart. Thinking back to my first few days in the army, when I had learned to swing a sledge hammer with precision, I carefully bashed the bottom ends of these timbers towards each other, until the beam was straight, and the king-post was properly seated. Next I built a concrete block wall under the beam, leaving a sizeable gap in the middle for the later installation of glazed doors. When it came time to remove the props, leaving the great beam supported by my new walls, I had visions of my precious concrete blocks collapsing, but all went well. I then removed the unsightly steel loop.

Another skill I had learned in the army was to 'wipe' soldered joints. This involved using a glove to spread the still just-molten solder over a joint in the lead covering of post office cables. Clearly I was a dab hand at soldering. So my next task was to install all the pipes we would need for the kitchen, the bathroom, two loos and the little shower room. I left the taps and other fittings to a proper plumber. And I did not attempt to install the electric pump we bought, for bringing water into the house from the well in our garden. Of course I had dealt with all manner of electrical jobs in the army. So yes, I put in all the cables, encased in their compulsory protective plastic tubes, leaving some of the fittings to an electrician to finish off, particularly the connections to the fuse box. After building the other walls downstairs, I got a builder to lay a concrete floor and to tile it. My pipes were hidden for ever. And then the builder plastered the walls – of course the unsightly wiring had vanished too.

On our next visit I built a staircase – what a good thing I had learned carpentry at school. With a lot of help from the family, I put in a first floor over half the building, the sitting/dining room taking up the other half, with the beautiful splay of timbers exposed to view – and the old beam ran at a level to make it ideal as a handrail for the landing. We had a proper front door fitted, four windows and French windows to what was to become the garden, and I made all the inside doors out of the very sensible French tongue-and-grooved floorboards. Then there were the timber and plasterboard walls to build upstairs. On each visit I rushed to work as soon as we arrived, and it was quite a wrench to go home again each time. This was clearly occupational therapy.

But the job did not end there. I put in some of the insulation of the roof, although I funked doing the biggest part – fifteen feet and more up in the sky. And I built my own solar heating panel on

148

the southern end of the building – that involved a lot more soldering. Eventually we left London and moved in. This meant that I had time to make a small workshop in an old chicken house, build a wood store and start the 'drinking platform' – and the garden. Mary had to admit that we were pretty comfortable. We even found time to have the odd evening drink outside – I was slacking!

One day, glass in hand, I spotted a slender shoot in the small flowerbed I had prepared just to one side. I had certainly not planted anything there yet. I discovered that it was an apricot tree. We had thrown the pips in that direction for a whole eating season. I moved it to a more suitable spot. Within four years it was producing literally hundreds of delicious apricots. At this stage I thought seriously of retiring properly. We had just had a garage built onto one end of the house, when I decided that what I really needed was a study. I had a builder put a French window in the back wall and then I partitioned off the rear quarter of the garage with those delightful French floorboards – it made a lovely study. I now had somewhere to keep my electronic concubine.

At some stage in this adventure we had a horrid shock. We were told to stop building, that we were in conflict with the planning authority. This was a real disaster. The previous owner had assured us that it would be all right. The lawyer dealing with our purchase had confirmed this. It transpired that both had known that no residential building was permitted in the locality. Not very good for the blood pressure! Happily we managed to sort everything out with the aid of the Mayor – then back to work.

After that I settled on reducing my occupational therapy – but not for long. My next venture into patienthood was the double vision I mentioned before. This demanded giving up driving, which meant that we had to move yet again – several miles each way for a loaf of bread was just not on. And, apart from the post, the only delivery we had to the shopless hamlet was olive oil every four weeks. Once more we were in a hurry.

The house we wanted was really too small for four of us. So we bought a tiny barn just round the corner as a sort of overflow. Then back to the occupational therapy with a vengeance. To start with we packed and unpacked seventy-four large cardboard boxes. The major improvements we left to a proper builder, who replaced the roof and the first floor of the barn and put in a new staircase and a loo. I was left to block up two doorways, put up innumerable bookshelves in the house and do a lot more in the barn. As soon as the roof and the rotten first floor of the barn had been replaced, I was at it again. I set up a small workshop on the ground floor, which also acted as store, while I panelled in the staircase and built a wardrobe upstairs, so that we could now have a spare room – just round the corner. I had annexed the spare room in the house as my study, so as to be within reach of the phone.

Unhappily this did not last very long. I was getting more and more breathless going uphill, and finally daughter and granddaughter returned to England. Yet another move was indicated – to a single-storey home, without hills. In the end we decided on a move halfway across France, where our elder son could keep and eye on us. Then back to the occupational therapy once more. Basil and a friend took out the garage door and replaced it with a French window. Next he laid a wood floor over the concrete, with very necessary insulation. Two-thirds of the way back we together built a wooden wall, leaving room for me to build yet another very small workshop. The front two thirds I panelled largely myself, again with excellent insulation, giving me a delightfully cosy small study. Basil then put a ceiling in. Happily there was a door from the old garage to the entrance hall, so I had access to the study without going out of the house. Of course, I still had shelves to put up. At last there was no more DIY to do. It seemed time for my third retirement.

I think back to the sad Lorna saying, 'My God, doctor, you've been there, too.' I have certainly experienced both sides of the 'medical divide'. There was so much I could no longer do. So what was left? My seventh medical book was just out – and here I was again writing in the non-medical field. I had read somewhere a delightful comment to the effect that 'writing a book is a minor marital infidelity'. I would sit long hours with my wonderful electronic playmate in what used to be the garage. She was so very much brighter than I was – and so much more up to date. She had truly known me in sickness and in health, and I certainly cherished her. But I still did not understand half of what she said. Thank heavens, in spite of this we certainly had a lot of highly therapeutic laughs together. Her name was 'Packard Bell' – *ma belle*.

MY ELECTRONIC CONCUBINE

Computer-illiterate, stupid or dumb,
You may label me just as you please.
Jack Horner was wiser, just stuck in his thumb,
And he ever remained at his ease.

I baulk at the jargon, I peer at my screen,
And I try to do everything right,
But I never remember the things that I've seen,
And I fail to do all that I might.

So what should I change in my concubine's house?
What on earth can I do to escape?
I gawk at the icons and play with my mouse,
And I have in my mind just one shape –

A pencil!

Then one more move – it had to be the last one. Two years after Mary's death I came back to England. More packing of boxes, more upheaval, necessary jettisoning of many chattels, more unpacking and finding places to put things. And yes, my small spare bedroom is inhabited by my electronic concubine. I could never have done it without the wonderful support of the family. Perhaps I have now really retired – time alone will tell.

11

The Quagmire – How May We Get Out Of it?

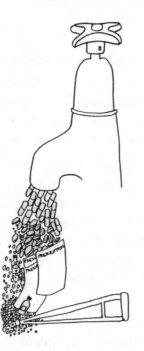

It was 22nd June 1947, It was a glorious day, with not a cloud to be seen. Looking from the window beside her bed in the maternity ward, Mary could see into the big room where I was sitting my anatomy examination. Margaret was just hatched – our very first baby and I had yet to see her. My exam paper handed in, I dashed up to see Mary and the new arrival. My reception was not quite what I had expected. She did not even mention the small pink parcel beside her.

'Hello, darling, I see you had a question on the shoulder.'

'How on earth did you know that?'

'That's easy. I could see some of the chaps waving their arms about in a very strange way. I soon realised that they were doing a sort of check-up on shoulder joint movements – don't forget I was a physiotherapist before I was a mum.'

So nothing was secret. And then I had a look at little Margaret. No surprises here, thank heavens. Soon Mary and Margaret would be at home and this would signal a new phase in my story. It was not long before I learned that I had passed the anatomy examination and was set to go on to the next stage as a clinical student. As mentioned earlier, this was the moment at which we ex-service students got into our stride in dealing with real live patients.

Apart from that episode and my twenty-sixth birthday, 1947 was notable for another reason. As a keen member of the hospital debating society, I was delighted to accept an invitation to second the opposition to a motion on the new White Paper outlining the government's proposals for setting up the National Health Service. The motion was proposed by a charming doctor who had chosen to defect from his profession to become an MP. I forget who seconded him. The motion was opposed by another doctor, who not very much later made a highly significant contribution to the advance of medical science. Before the meeting I read the White Paper carefully, noting a number of oddities, including several unsupported claims and wild predictions. On the evening of the debate I had a short discussion with the doctor I was to support. We agreed on a low-key approach, discreetly questioning some of the predictions made. The debate proved lively, and we managed to convince the house that the White Paper was not at all satisfactory. The motion was well and truly lost. I was of course delighted, but I did not expect anything further to come out of that rather stimulating evening. I was wrong.

Days later I had another invitation – to join the Fellowship for Freedom in Medicine. I became the only student member. This was the start of a most interesting short period, during which a very serious group of dedicated doctors looked at every proposal in the White Paper, putting together a discussion document for presentation to the Minister of Health. They were making a serious bid to improve the proposed service, for the good of their patients. One of the doctors involved was not only a doctor, he had also qualified as a barrister, in addition to which he had been an MP for a number of years. Very quiet and gentle in manner, whenever he spoke at a meeting everyone listened intently. He said what he thought – and clearly first thought about what he was going to say. This habit had earlier triggered his political downfall. He was intelligent, widely educated, thoughtful, honest and fearless. His party, apparently more interested in allegiance to party politics than sober consideration of social problems, found him an embarrassment, although most of his constituents respected him greatly. Failing to persuade him to abandon his honest approach, his party went to the extent of attempting to get him certified as of unsound mind. This is not a joke – it is true. It did little to enhance my pretty dim view of politics and politicians. He was well out of it – but people like him were surely needed.

The Minister of Health agreed rather reluctantly to meet a small delegation from the Fellowship for Freedom in Medicine. Whether or not he had bothered to read our carefully prepared discussion document was not clear. What rapidly did become clear was that Aneurin Bevan chose to be extremely rude to this group of serious, dedicated doctors, dismissing everything they said out of hand and accusing them of self-interest and greed. It is of note that over the next few years every one of the predictions we made came true. My view of politicians sank even lower. But there was far worse to come.

As had appeared in the hospital debate, the medical profession was divided in its views on the proposed NHS. The majority was not really persuaded that this was the best way to solve the very real social problems that existed before and after the war. After all, Lord Beveridge had defined in his earlier report the serious economic factors threatening society. I understood them well, as I had grown up with them. Bevan chose to ignore any suggestion that basically economic problems might best be addressed by economic solutions. He demanded social revolution. If the medical profession chose to be difficult, he would divide them before imposing his will on them and on the people.

In the months that followed, Bevan made use of two quite odious strategies to get his way. At first failing to satisfy the British Medical Association or the Royal Colleges of his wisdom, he proposed a system of secret merit awards which would be available to an appreciable number of those specialists who toed his line, which could result in increasing their earnings by up to one hundred per cent. (And of course this would be reflected in their pensions.) There is but one word for this – and it is nothing to laugh about – bribery. And the wretched man even bragged publicly that he had 'stuffed their mouths with gold'. Bevan's words, not mine. He was actually proud of his disgraceful behaviour. The gold of obedience seemed charged with a smell nothing to do with holiness – it just stank.

Many general practitioners were unconvinced, too. In dealing with them, Bevan's position was greatly aided by the comment of a very senior specialist, who publicly referred to general practitioners as those doctors who had 'fallen off the ladder of success'. Words like this coming from a senior medical figure must have been music to Bevan's ear. He determined to squash any rebellion from these second-class doctors. He knew well that a substantial proportion of them had had to borrow money to purchase the goodwill in their practices. This they had accepted without question – it was a long-term investment, made worthwhile by their independence and reasonable security. The new bill made the purchase and sale of goodwill in the practice illegal, from the date of initiation of the service. But Bevan's real master stroke was to impose a time limit for general practitioners to 'sign on' in the NHS. A doctor not signing his contract by the due date would forfeit for ever any right to recoup the capital he had invested. Almost as an afterthought, Bevan further decreed that even those who did sign on prior to the due date would not have their investment refunded until they retired. And no interest would be payable in the meantime, either.

Happily for me, because of my six years' war service, I was still a medical student, so I was spared being put in this impossible situation. But it meant that many of those already in practice would continue to pay interest on loans that had been effectively confiscated by the State. Again no laughing matter – this was nothing short of blackmail. Bevan's behaviour was quite despicable. Bribery and blackmail prevailed. He won the day – on a political platform.

The great majority of the medical profession set about trying their best to make a seriously flawed system work effectively – for their patients. But their task was to be made more and more difficult as the years passed, and as more and more politically prompted changes were inflicted upon them. Of course, every change demanded more and more time being spent *not* looking after their patients, and more and more administrative staff to edge the NHS steadily towards bankruptcy. No laughs at all on this point.

The NHS was only three and a half years old when I entered rural general practice. The two of us then in the practice did very nearly all our own dispensing. We were happy to take on this additional task for our patients, as the nearest pharmacist was ten miles from the practice centre, and most patients had no transport beyond a bicycle. One of the very early administrative idiocies I met personally was the imposition of prescription charges. I remember it well. The original charge was one shilling per item. Of course, some patients were exempt from payment of the charge. These included retired patients over a certain age, children under a certain age and expectant mothers. No, I was not required to produce certified copies of birth certificates or evidence of pregnancy.

But what really happened? From those not in these three categories I was required to take one shilling for each item dispensed. That was easy – it went into my trouser pocket. Occasionally there was a problem in finding the right change. I then had to waste more time sticking a one-shilling postage stamp on a special form. This form had been devised and produced (at some wholly unnecessary expense to the taxpayer) to provide space for twenty stamps, each one of which had to be franked. On completion of one form I had to fill in practice details, date it, sign it and put it to one side until the end of the month. Then I had to gather the forms together, count them, enter the score on yet another specially produced form and send the lot to the appropriate administrative body. Whether anyone looked at the forms remains untold, and certainly there was no way in which such scrutiny could have helped a solitary patient. Of course there was no means of telling whether I had collected the right number of shillings, either. What was clear was that I had to spend an appreciable amount of time each month *not* looking after my patients.

How much time? Suppose I saw thirty patients per day and that, on average, each one needed only one prescription – and that is a modest estimate. This would involve going to the post office several times each month to buy 900 one-shilling stamps, tearing them one by one from the sheet, licking them, sticking them in their little squares, scribbling on 46 sheets of wasted paper, and sending the package to the authority concerned. The only laugh to be had is at the crass idiocy of such an administrative cock-up. It could only add to our frustration and be to our patients' disadvantage – in addition to costing money better spent on doing something useful for the patients.

This was more than half a century ago. Every year since has been marked by some administrative change in the service – there would certainly be no laughs if I were to detail them all. But they do demand comment with regard to their cumulative results. Perhaps we may start with a real laugh? Bevan's original estimate of the cost of the whole NHS was 19 million pounds per annum – but even more ludicrous, he solemnly predicted that this sum would *decrease* as the health of the nation improved. Who did he think he was kidding? Yes, one of the things the FFM had told him was that this was no more than a dream – that the reverse would prove true, probably in quite a big way.

I have long thought it ridiculous to speak of professional boxers or footballers. They are *commercial* boxers or footballers –

sometimes to great effect – and the best of luck to them. The priesthood, the law, medicine, dentistry and teaching are a few examples of true professions. What makes them different? Each is based on a required educational curriculum. Every entrant has to provide evidence of having achieved a minimum standard of competence. Every professional is bound to practise within well-defined rules of procedure. In each case there exists a monitoring system with disciplinary powers. And very proper too. When it comes to politicians, there is no specific education for the job, there are no standards of competence to be met, there is little to define how they should behave. Apart from ridding Parliament of them (by fair means or foul) there is no control mechanism – other than what the party chiefs or their financial supporters demand. No, not by any stretch of the imagination are politicians professionals.

I welcome one improvement since 1951. At that time my basic rate of pay for seeing a patient, either in the surgery or at home, night or day, worked out at twelve and a half old pence. That must be good cause for a laugh, a professional fee of twelve and a half pence. Even for those who had 'fallen off the ladder of success', this was derisory, no less than an affront. What did I do? I did my best for my patients – under more and more difficult circumstances. Happily the rewards got quite a lot better after a while, though not before time.

I seem to be indulging in an unending moan. But it is necessary to have a grasp of the history of the NHS if we are to salvage it from the ghastly havoc that the politicians have wreaked. What havoc? Perhaps we may start with the reduction in the overall number of hospital beds available to our patients, the unacceptably long waits for appointments and admissions, the closure of whole hospitals, passing the buck to others because the doctor is busy at an administrative meeting or attempting to meet illusory targets, rather than dealing with his patients. (There was one occasion when five million pounds was spent on building a new hospital block, only to have it closed within two or three years because the body in charge could not afford the cost of maintaining it.) Then there have been countless changes in systems of payment, each causing unnecessary, frustrating and costly upheaval.

We seem overdue for a laugh. So it might be well to look at an illustration of just how idiotic the situation could be. A good many years ago, as in the eyes of our non-professional masters partnerships in general practice were not good enough, it was decided that group practices should be encouraged. Bigger was better. Merger mania had taken over. The clever fellows ordained the award of group practice allowances – yes, something approaching bribery again – for amalgamating previously independent practices, whether they were operating effectively or not.

By this time there were three of us in partnership, operating from three centres strung out along the Great North Road four or five miles from each other. We duly applied for our allowance. It was refused (by the appropriate, inevitably non-professional committee) on the grounds that we were not all three operating from a single, central building. When we pointed out that doing so would greatly inconvenience two-thirds of our patients, the administrators were unmoved – they were not even slightly interested in the quality of care offered. They were intent upon implementing the new allowance whether it helped patients or hindered them.

It was Maurice who came up with our answer. If we were to dissolve the partnership and work as three single-handed practices we would each qualify for a single-handed practice allowance. Yes, that is what we did – and three single-handed practice allowances were just about as much as the one group practice allowance we had been denied. Of course our patients were delighted not to have to travel miles out of their way. We were able to maintain our standard of service and continued to work as a well-coordinated team, while no longer being in formal partnership. Legally binding partnership was replaced by mutual trust – and it worked very well for many years.

This sort of unnecessary, senseless change, year after year, has had several serious effects. First it has wasted more and more professional time, which should have been devoted to the care of patients. Second it has increased the administrative cost of the service at every turn – paid not by the government, but by the long-suffering taxpayer. Third it has gradually worn down the spirit of the medical profession, resulting in more and more applications for early retirement, with fewer and fewer new faces seeking to take their places. And now, largely because the administrators have failed to keep to their budgets, we have piecemeal privatisation of services. Of course it is only proper for a private company to make a profit – so the result of this new lunacy can only be to further increase the cost. Today Ministers of Health sometimes appear to be as ill-informed about medicine and as uninterested in the patients' welfare as Bevan was.

So what about the needs and desires of patients? They are the ones who should count most. As described earlier, I write as an experienced patient. I would very much prefer never to see a doctor again, let alone be admitted to hospital. I accept this to be an impossible dream. So back to reality.

If I do need help, I want to see a properly trained, qualified individual – a person whom I can get to know and trust – an individual who knows me and respects me as a person. I want to see a true professional. I do not want to be passed to someone who may be able to help, with no proper assessment in the first place. Of course my doctor will have his shortcomings – with today's rate of change in medical science, he will certainly not know everything – but one thing he will know is fundamental. He will know where to find all the information he seeks – there it is, sitting on his desk inside his computer, much of it even in the palm of his hand. More important still, he will know how to weigh the facts he extracts from the appropriate website. The third thing he will know is how best to interpret those facts he elicits – for each patient – and such explanation must be worded very differently when offered to a farmer, a dressmaker or a Professor of Medieval History.

As I know from long experience wearing my professional hat, it is easy enough to 'get it wrong' with the patient in the consulting room – within sight, hearing and touch. The risk of error can only be increased by discarding any of these three – the telephone consultation may be superficially convenient, it may even be cheaper at the time, but it is fundamentally dangerous – the risk of 'getting it wrong' is inevitably increased. I do not want that when I need help. Yet only very recently the Royal College of General Practitioners has published a small book on the subject. Similarly, if I choose to go to the medical supermarket or visit various websites on my own, the risk is again increased (unless I have a sound, up-to-date professional understanding of the subject) – and any unfavourable result is therefore my fault. Not for me, thank you.

What of referral to a specialist? I want three things in this respect. For a start I want my doctor to point me in the right direction – first time. He is more likely to achieve this if he has plenty of time to see me, rather than dashing past between administrative meetings or desperately trying to meet unrealistic targets. Second I want to see the chosen specialist within days of referral. As in the case of writing a letter, the consultation takes no longer today than it will in three months' time, or more. Only recently has a distinguished specialist declared that, due to administrative demands, he is able to spend no more than half his working day in the presence of patients. This is shocking. Third I want any necessary hospitalisation to be made available promptly and conducted to high professional standards. I do not want four-star hotel rating, neither do I want to be 'put on the back burner' because I am of an age some non-professional nerd says is worthy of neglect.

The sad thing is that this dream would have been possible if Bevan had taken the Fellowship for Freedom in Medicine seriously all those years ago – at a truly gigantic saving to the taxpayer. It is not the medical profession who have failed the patients, it is the fundamentally unworkable system thrust upon us by truly non-professional politicians – only to suffer administrative and organisational change over and over again.

And now we learn that the NHS is the third largest employer in the world, yet the percentage of this enormous army actually helping patients is pitifully small. Again no laughter. I wish you could wake up from this horrid nightmare, the laughs I have recorded in previous chapters still ringing in your ears. The costly hordes of administrators are gone, the ill-trained, gold-driven politicians have relinquished their stinking stranglehold on the medical profession, and you are sitting in peace with your trusted family doctor. Well, anyone can dream!

As the Fellowship for Freedom in Medicine told Bevan all those years ago, what we have needed all along is a simple, impersonal National Health Insurance Plan, with no intrusion of political or administrative concerns into the highly personal relationship we may once again enjoy with a dedicated profession. When you wake up, you might well speak to your MP. Surely that could provoke the last laugh – he or she will probably not know a thing about the subject.

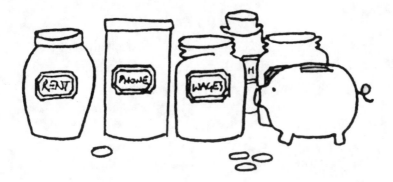